Pills and Politics

Americans' Struggle for Affordable Medication

Douglas B Sims, PhD

Douglas B Sims

Pills and Politics

Copyright © 2024 by Douglas B. Sims

All rights reserved. No part of this book may be used or reproduced in any form whatsoever without written permission except in the case of brief quotations in critical articles or reviews.

Printed in the United States of America.

For more information, or to book an event, contact:
dsims@simsassociates.net

Book design by DB Sims
Cover picture: George Robinson, iStock

ISBN – Paperback: 979-8-9919108-0-4
ISBN – eBook: 979-8-9919108-1-1

First Edition: October 2024

Douglas B Sims

Table of Contents

Acknowledgements vii
Forward ix
1. The Cost of Health 1
2. A Historical Perspective 4
3. How Drugs Are Priced 12
4. Government and Price Regulation 21
5. The Role of Patents and Generic Drugs 28
6. Lobbying and Political Influence 35
7. Direct-to-Consumer Advertising 41
8. The Impact on Patients and Healthcare Systems 48
9. Alternatives to the American System 54
10. Attempts at Reform in the U.S. 62
11. Possible Solutions for America 69
12. Why Democrats nor Republicans Will Ever Fix Drug Prices 78
13. Big Pharma and Insurance Companies 88
14. The Future of Prescription Drug Pricing 97
Bibliography 102
About the Author 110
Glossary of Key Terms 111
Legislative Timeline 113

Douglas B Sims

Acknowledgements

I want to extend my heartfelt gratitude to my wife for her steadfast support, wisdom, and the extraordinary journey of love and partnership we've shared over the past 34 years. You have been my anchor and inspiration through life and this entire process.

I am equally grateful to our two children, who have filled our lives with joy and growth, teaching us the rewards and trials of parenthood. Watching you grow has been a constant source of pride and valuable lessons.

To our family: Thank you for walking alongside us and offering unwavering support. Your companionship and encouragement have been invaluable.

I am profoundly grateful to my friends and colleagues, especially health professionals and political scientists, with whom I've had the privilege to discuss, debate, and explore complex ideas. Your perspectives, expertise, and insights have greatly enriched the depth and authenticity of this book, making this journey both enlightening and rewarding.

I also extend my appreciation to the many individuals I've had the opportunity to observe and interact with across various professional settings. Your experiences and contributions have provided invaluable insights, adding layers of real-world understanding and perspective to these pages. Thank you all for your role in this endeavor.

Douglas B Sims

Forward

This book delves into the world of high-cost pharmaceuticals in the United States, examining the complex web of industry practices, political dependencies, and structural barriers that drive drug prices ever higher, placing an immense burden on American patients. At its core, the issue goes beyond mere economics—it's a system built on policies and incentives that allow costs to rise unchecked, without sufficient safeguards for the public.

Despite widespread support for reform, both major political parties—Republicans and Democrats—are unlikely to implement the transformative changes needed. Their dependency on campaign contributions from pharmaceutical companies and industry lobbyists creates a powerful disincentive to challenge this broken system. As a result, the status quo remains firmly in place, where both parties benefit from Big Pharma's contributions, leaving consumers to shoulder the financial burden.

Consequently, Americans disproportionately bear the cost of high drug prices, essentially subsidizing more affordable access to medications in other parts of the world. While citizens in other nations benefit from government-regulated pricing and cost controls, U.S. patients pay some of the highest prices globally. This disparity allows Big Pharma to rake in billions on the backs of Americans, while charging significantly less in countries where governments prioritize citizens' health over industry profits. In contrast, American politicians, often more focused on securing their next election and reliant on industry donations, fall short in addressing the long-term health and financial security of their constituents.

For meaningful change, the United States can draw valuable lessons from other countries that have successfully balanced innovation, affordability, and access. Policies that introduce government-led price negotiations, streamline pathways for generics and biosimilars, and enforce transparency in drug pricing could provide a pathway toward a more equitable system.

The future of prescription drug pricing in America requires unified action from all stakeholders—policymakers, healthcare providers, and the public. Policymakers must champion legislation that prioritizes patient access; healthcare providers need to advocate for affordable treatment options; and patients themselves are crucial advocates for change, driving grassroots movements that remind leaders of the urgent need for reform.

Though the journey toward a fairer, more affordable healthcare system is complex, the stakes are too high to ignore. By confronting the forces that inflate drug prices and championing reforms that prioritize public health, there is real potential to reshape the pharmaceutical landscape. The time for change is now—through commitment, collaboration, and informed action, the promise of affordable healthcare for all Americans can become a reality.

Chapter 1

The Cost of Health: How Prescription Prices Shape Lives

Prescription drug prices in the United States have become a major burden for many Americans, influencing not only their financial stability but also their access to necessary healthcare. The problem of inflated prescription costs is multifaceted, driven by a combination of regulatory gaps, economic structures, and corporate power. In comparison to other developed countries, particularly in Europe, the U.S. stands out for its disproportionately high pharmaceutical prices, which can be attributed to the unique system in which drug prices are determined.

In the U.S., there is no centralized mechanism to negotiate drug prices at the federal level, which contrasts sharply with the price control systems employed in the European Union (EU) and other developed nations. In Europe, governments typically negotiate directly with pharmaceutical companies, setting maximum prices and ensuring that the cost of medicines remains affordable for the population (Wouters et al., 2020). In the U.S., however, pharmaceutical companies are free to set prices independently, often leading to extreme markups for critical medications such as insulin, cancer treatments, and life-saving antibiotics (Sarnak et al., 2017). This laissez-faire approach to drug pricing has resulted in Americans paying more per capita on prescription drugs than citizens of any other country (OECD, 2022).

This issue has wide-reaching consequences for both individual patients and the overall economy. For many Americans, the cost of medications forces them to make difficult choices between healthcare and other essential expenses. A survey by the Kaiser Family Foundation found that nearly 29% of Americans report not taking their medications as prescribed because of the high costs (KFF, 2019). This lack of adherence can lead to worse health outcomes, increased hospitalizations, and higher long-term healthcare costs, which further strain the system.

At the macroeconomic level, high drug prices contribute to rising healthcare expenditures, which now account for nearly 18% of the U.S. GDP (Centers for Medicare & Medicaid Services, 2022). This not only impacts the federal budget but also the private sector, where employers are forced to shoulder increasing healthcare costs for their employees. As pharmaceutical costs escalate, they also drive up insurance premiums, co-pays, and out-of-pocket expenses for consumers, exacerbating economic inequality and reducing access to care for lower-income populations (Anderson et al., 2019).

Three key factors underpin the prescription drug price problem in the U.S.: regulation, economics, and corporate influence. First, the lack of governmental price controls contrasts sharply with the strategies employed in Europe, where regulatory frameworks enforce price ceilings and incentivize the use of generic drugs (Morgan et al., 2017). Second, the economic structures in the U.S., where the market is driven by profit-seeking behavior, have enabled pharmaceutical companies to monopolize the market for extended periods due to strong patent protections, delaying the introduction of cheaper generic alternatives (Kesselheim et al., 2018). Finally, the political influence of pharmaceutical companies through lobbying and campaign contributions has hampered meaningful reform efforts, allowing drug prices to remain artificially high (Taylor et al., 2019).

Addressing the prescription drug price crisis is essential for improving the health of the American population and ensuring the sustainability of the U.S. healthcare system. As this book will explore, the solution lies in understanding the complex web of regulatory, economic, and corporate factors that have led to the current state of affairs. By examining how other developed countries have successfully managed their drug prices, the U.S. can begin to reform its policies and create a system where life-saving medications are accessible to all, without the burden of exorbitant costs.

Chapter 2

A Historical Perspective

The rise of Big Pharma in America is a story of unprecedented growth, strategic consolidation, and the entrenchment of corporate power in one of the world's most profitable industries. Over the past century, the U.S. pharmaceutical industry has transformed from small, family-owned businesses producing basic medicines into a multibillion-dollar global enterprise. This transformation was driven not only by scientific advancements but also by a unique regulatory and economic environment that allowed pharmaceutical companies to dominate the market, shape drug prices, and exert significant influence over healthcare policy. Unlike Europe, where government intervention in healthcare costs is the norm, the U.S. adopted a market-driven approach, allowing Big Pharma to flourish with minimal oversight. This chapter traces the evolution of the U.S. pharmaceutical industry, the regulatory frameworks that enabled its rise, the role of patents in maintaining market exclusivity, and the impact of direct-to-consumer advertising, a distinctly American practice that has further entrenched the power and profitability of these corporations.

The Rise of Big Pharma in America

The evolution of the pharmaceutical industry in the United States is a narrative of transformation, from modest 19th-century origins to an industry that is today both a global leader in medical innovation and a formidable force in shaping healthcare policy and pricing. Early pharmaceutical companies were small, often family-run businesses producing basic medicines. However, by the 20th century, significant advances in chemistry and medicine, coupled with government investments and collaborations, propelled the industry into a new era of drug discovery and production. This growth was fueled not only by scientific progress but also by strategic mergers and acquisitions, which allowed a few large corporations to consolidate resources, knowledge, and market control.

A critical driver of the industry's dominance is its unique regulatory environment, which diverges sharply from the models found in European countries. In the U.S., regulations initially aimed at protecting public health gradually adapted to support pharmaceutical innovation and commercialization, allowing companies to recoup research costs by setting prices with minimal government interference. Unlike European healthcare systems, where governments negotiate prices or impose caps, U.S. policy favored free-market principles. The patent system also played a major role in cementing the industry's power. Strong patent protections enabled pharmaceutical companies to maintain monopolies on new drugs, delaying the introduction of generic alternatives and allowing companies to set high prices during the patent period, a strategy rarely seen in Europe, where patents and price controls balance more evenly.

The introduction of direct-to-consumer (DTC) advertising in the 1980s marked another turning point, creating a uniquely American phenomenon that boosted the visibility and profitability of pharmaceutical companies. DTC advertising—only fully permitted in the U.S. and New Zealand—allowed companies to market directly to patients, encouraging them to request specific drugs from their healthcare providers. This shift not only increased demand but also reshaped the doctor-patient relationship, placing consumers in a more active role while reinforcing the pharmaceutical industry's reach and influence.

In examining the historical development of the U.S. pharmaceutical industry, this chapter will explore how these factors—the regulatory environment, patent protections, consolidation, and DTC advertising—collectively differentiated the U.S. model from European approaches. This unique combination of elements has allowed American pharmaceutical companies to wield unprecedented power over drug pricing and consumer behavior, shaping the landscape of healthcare in ways that continue to reverberate globally.

The Evolution of the Pharmaceutical Industry in the U.S.

The origins of the U.S. pharmaceutical industry date back to the 19th century when small, family-owned businesses produced patent medicines, which were often unregulated and marketed as cure-alls despite their limited efficacy (Hirsch, 2021). These early medicines, advertised with bold claims but lacking rigorous testing, laid the foundation for an industry that would later undergo significant transformation. By the early 20th century, scientific breakthroughs, including the discoveries of penicillin and insulin, began to reshape the pharmaceutical landscape. This era marked a shift toward research-driven drug development, with companies now focusing on the discovery and production of scientifically validated medicines (Scherer, 2019).

The post-World War II period accelerated this shift, ushering in a time of unprecedented growth for the industry. With antibiotics, vaccines, and other life-saving treatments emerging, companies such as Pfizer, Merck, and Eli Lilly established themselves as leaders in medical innovation. This period saw pharmaceutical firms investing heavily in research and development (R&D), a strategy that laid the groundwork for the era of "blockbuster drugs." These high-revenue products dominated the market for years, generating immense profits and establishing these companies as global powerhouses in the industry.

Strategic mergers and acquisitions further fueled the industry's expansion, allowing pharmaceutical giants to consolidate resources, enhance R&D capabilities, and broaden their market reach. This consolidation not only strengthened the financial position of these companies but also increased their influence in shaping drug pricing and healthcare policies. By the late 20th century, the U.S. pharmaceutical industry had evolved into a dominant force on the global stage, with American companies consistently ranking among the top producers of prescription drugs worldwide (Rosenberg, 2019).

This transformation—from small, unregulated businesses to global leaders in medical innovation—reflects the powerful interplay of scientific progress, strategic corporate growth, and an evolving regulatory environment. As the industry expanded, these elements collectively set the stage for the emergence of a uniquely American pharmaceutical model, one that would later grapple with complex challenges related to drug pricing, market influence, and healthcare accessibility.

The 20th-Century Regulatory Environment and Patent Laws

The regulatory environment in the U.S. has been instrumental in shaping the pharmaceutical industry's development, establishing a framework that prioritizes both drug safety and industry innovation. The 1906 Pure Food and Drug Act marked the federal government's first major step to regulate the safety and efficacy of drugs, responding to public concerns over fraudulent health claims and unsafe medicines (Carpenter, 2014). This law laid the groundwork for more comprehensive drug regulation, which was further strengthened by the 1938 Food, Drug, and Cosmetic Act. This act required that new drugs be tested for safety before being marketed to consumers, expanding federal oversight and setting a precedent for rigorous testing standards (Hutt & Merrill, 2020).

The establishment of the U.S. Food and Drug Administration (FDA) in 1930 marked a turning point, as the agency became responsible for enforcing drug regulations and safeguarding public health. Later amendments, such as the 1962 Kefauver-Harris Drug Amendments, reinforced the FDA's role, requiring proof of both safety and efficacy for all new drugs. These amendments were spurred by the thalidomide tragedy, where a sedative prescribed to pregnant women resulted in thousands of birth defects. The FDA's expanded authority allowed it to implement more stringent drug approval processes, which became the global gold standard for pharmaceutical oversight (FDA, 2022).

In addition to regulatory oversight, patent law has been a key driver of the pharmaceutical industry's growth. Under the U.S. patent system, pharmaceutical companies receive exclusive rights to produce and sell new drugs for up to 20 years from the patent application date, allowing them to recoup the high costs associated with research and development (Kesselheim et al., 2018). This exclusivity is essential for companies to profit from their innovations before facing competition from generic alternatives. However, the extensive patent protection period has also contributed to high drug prices, especially when combined with practices like "evergreening." Through evergreening, companies make minor changes to existing drugs—such as altering dosage or delivery methods—to extend patent protection, thereby delaying generic competition and maintaining high prices (Hemphill & Sampat, 2012).

In contrast, European countries often employ shorter patent protection periods and enforce stricter rules against evergreening, enabling generic drugs to enter the market sooner and at lower costs (Morgan et al., 2017). This regulatory difference has contributed to the comparatively high prices seen in the U.S., where prolonged exclusivity and limited price control measures allow companies to maintain elevated pricing for longer.

Together, the U.S. regulatory environment and patent system have cultivated a pharmaceutical industry characterized by innovation and profit but also by significant challenges related to accessibility and affordability. As this chapter will explore, understanding the regulatory and legal frameworks that govern the industry is crucial to addressing the complex issue of drug pricing and finding a sustainable path forward for American healthcare.

How U.S. Healthcare and Pharmaceutical Systems Developed Differently from Europe

The development of the U.S. healthcare and pharmaceutical systems diverged sharply from Europe, driven by contrasting ideologies around government intervention and market regulation. In the mid-20th century, many European nations established universal healthcare systems, a framework designed to treat healthcare as a public good rather than a commercial enterprise. In these systems, government entities play a central role in regulating healthcare costs, including prescription drug prices, to ensure broad access. By negotiating directly with pharmaceutical companies, European governments leverage their purchasing power to establish maximum prices, securing more affordable medications for their populations (Wouters et al., 2020). This approach reflects a broader commitment to ensuring that healthcare remains accessible to all citizens, with affordability prioritized over corporate profit margins.

In contrast, the U.S. opted for a market-driven healthcare model, with limited government control over prescription drug pricing. The U.S. system relies heavily on private insurance, which has evolved alongside a profit-centered pharmaceutical industry. This industry model prioritizes shareholder returns and profitability, leading to a structure where pharmaceutical companies determine drug prices based on market demand and potential profitability, rather than government-imposed price ceilings (Anderson et al., 2019). Although the FDA oversees drug safety and efficacy, it does not regulate drug pricing. As a result, pharmaceutical companies in the U.S. can set prices independently, often leading to significantly higher drug costs than in Europe (Squires et al., 2017).

This divergence in healthcare models reflects fundamentally different views on healthcare access and affordability. While European countries see healthcare as a right that necessitates government intervention to protect citizens from unaffordable costs, the U.S. model places healthcare within a free-market system where accessibility can be secondary to profitability. This approach has led to a pharmaceutical system in the U.S. where profits frequently overshadow accessibility, contributing to today's crisis of high drug prices and limited affordability for many Americans.

The Introduction of Direct-to-Consumer Drug Advertising in the U.S.

One of the most striking differences between the U.S. and other countries, particularly in Europe, is the practice of direct-to-consumer (DTC) drug advertising. In 1997, the FDA relaxed its regulations on pharmaceutical advertising, allowing companies to market prescription drugs directly to consumers via television, radio, and print media (Ventola, 2011). The U.S. and New Zealand are the only two countries where DTC advertising is legal, and the impact on drug pricing has been profound.

Pharmaceutical companies spend billions of dollars each year on advertising, promoting drugs for conditions ranging from high cholesterol to erectile dysfunction (Donohue et al., 2007). This marketing strategy has led to increased demand for brand-name drugs, even when cheaper generic alternatives are available. Critics argue that DTC advertising misleads consumers by promoting drugs as quick fixes for complex health problems while downplaying potential side effects (Mintzes et al., 2019). Moreover, the cost of advertising is often passed on to consumers through higher drug prices. In contrast, European countries have banned or heavily restricted DTC advertising, focusing instead on educating healthcare providers, who serve as gatekeepers for prescribing medications (Wouters et al., 2020). This difference in approach has helped keep drug costs lower in Europe and prevented the kind of overprescription that has become common in the U.S.

In summary, the rise of Big Pharma in America is a story of regulatory evolution, economic strategy, and corporate dominance. Unlike their European counterparts, U.S. pharmaceutical companies operate in a largely unregulated pricing environment, protected by strong patent laws and fueled by aggressive marketing strategies. The introduction of DTC advertising further entrenched the power of Big

Pharma, creating a system where drug prices continue to rise, leaving millions of Americans struggling to afford life-saving medications. Understanding this historical context is crucial for developing meaningful reforms that can address the root causes of the U.S. prescription drug crisis.

Chapter 3

How Drugs Are Priced

Pharmaceutical pricing is a complex and multi-layered process shaped by various factors, ranging from research and development (R&D) costs to the regulatory environment and market competition. Unlike typical consumer goods, drug prices are not determined solely by production expenses or standard supply-and-demand dynamics. Instead, pharmaceutical companies account for the significant financial and time investments required to develop, test, and secure regulatory approval for new drugs. This process, which can span over a decade, includes the high costs associated with extensive clinical trials, compliance with regulatory requirements, and the acquisition of patents that grant market exclusivity. These patent protections allow companies to recover development costs by setting prices without competition from generics for a set period.

Beyond these direct costs, the structure of the pharmaceutical supply chain itself contributes to the final price paid by consumers. Intermediaries such as pharmacy benefit managers (PBMs), insurers, and wholesalers each play a role in determining price markups, negotiating rebates, and setting formulary placements. While these intermediaries are intended to manage costs and provide accessibility, their involvement can add layers to the pricing structure that often lead to higher out-of-pocket expenses for consumers.

This chapter delves into the intricate factors that shape drug pricing, including the protective role of patents, the high costs and risks associated with clinical trials, and the exclusivity periods granted by regulatory agencies. Additionally, we explore the strategies pharmaceutical companies use to price drugs based on factors like therapeutic value, market competition, and the demographics of the patient population. By dissecting these elements, we gain a clearer understanding of why drug prices vary so widely between countries and why access to affordable medications continues to be a global challenge. Through this exploration, we uncover the economic, regulatory, and ethical considerations that make drug pricing a critical issue for both patients and healthcare systems worldwide: the tables below show the process by which drug prices are set in the USA and the EU:

Drug Pricing in the USA

Factor	Description
Market-Driven Pricing	Pharmaceutical companies set drug prices based on market demand and competition, with limited direct regulation on initial pricing.
Patent Exclusivity	New drugs receive patent protection (typically 20 years from filing), allowing companies to maintain high prices without generic competition.
Pharmacy Benefit Managers	PBMs negotiate rebates with manufacturers to place drugs on formularies, but rebates are often not passed directly to consumers.
Medicare & Medicaid	Medicare cannot negotiate prices directly with manufacturers, though Medicaid receives mandated rebates on covered drugs.
DTC Advertising Costs	High costs for direct-to-consumer advertising contribute to drug prices; U.S. is one of the few countries allowing DTC pharmaceutical ads.
Research & Development	Drug prices reflect recovery of R&D costs, though actual R&D spending vs. profit ratios are often debated.
Lack of Price Transparency	Manufacturers are not required to disclose pricing calculations, making it challenging for consumers to understand price breakdowns.
No National Price Regulation	No centralized body sets or limits drug prices; prices are generally set by the manufacturer and influenced by market competition.

Drug Pricing in the European Union

Factor	Description
Regulated Price Controls	Many EU countries have governmental or independent agencies that set or cap drug prices to ensure affordability.
Health Technology Assessment (HTA)	Drugs undergo HTA processes to evaluate their cost-effectiveness and impact on public health, influencing reimbursement and price setting.
Reference Pricing System	Drug prices are often compared to those in other EU countries, with reference pricing used to set or negotiate costs at a standardized level.
Negotiated Discounts	Governments negotiate directly with manufacturers for discounts or rebates, allowing for lower prices for public healthcare systems.
Pharmaceutical Price Regulation	Each country's health system regulates prices, particularly for reimbursable medicines, limiting price increases post-launch.
Patent & Exclusivity Protections	Patent protections exist, but many EU nations encourage rapid entry of generics post-exclusivity to foster competition and reduce prices.
No DTC Advertising	Direct-to-consumer pharmaceutical advertising is generally prohibited, limiting marketing costs in drug pricing.
Transparency Requirements	EU regulations require price transparency in many cases, with some nations requiring manufacturers to justify price hikes based on costs.

The Economics Behind Prescription Costs

Prescription drug prices in the United States are notably higher than those in most other developed nations, often placing a severe financial strain on American consumers seeking life-saving medications (see table below). Drug pricing in the U.S. is driven by a complex web of factors, including the substantial costs of research and development (R&D), patent protections that grant monopolies, limited market competition, and the profit-driven nature of the industry. Together, these factors have created an environment where drug costs are set according to what the market will tolerate, rather than being tightly regulated.

One of the primary economic strategies behind high drug prices in the U.S. is the recovery of R&D expenditures. Pharmaceutical companies invest heavily in developing new medications, a process that includes years of research, clinical trials, and regulatory approvals. The industry often argues that high prices are necessary to recoup these costs, yet R&D expenses vary widely by drug, and high prices are often maintained long after R&D investments have been recovered. Additionally, patent monopolies grant companies exclusive rights to produce and sell a new drug for up to 20 years, limiting competition and enabling higher prices during this period.

Medication	US ($)	UK ($)	France ($)	Canada ($)	Mexico ($)	Argentina ($)	Japan ($)	Australia ($)
Atorvastatin	0.97	0.39	0.53	0.93	0.55	0.36	0.56	0.85
Lisinopril	0.07	0.13	0.21	0.07	0.08	0.06	0.28	0.10
Levothyroxine	0.30	0.26	0.16	0.26	0.19	0.11	0.21	0.26
Metformin	0.15	0.07	0.08	0.15	0.06	0.05	0.35	0.14
Amlodipine	0.14	0.08	0.11	0.11	0.07	0.05	0.42	0.12
Simvastatin	0.23	0.16	0.16	0.22	0.10	0.08	0.49	0.16
Omeprazole	0.57	0.45	0.47	0.48	0.22	0.17	0.63	0.39
Gabapentin	0.36	0.26	0.26	0.30	0.14	0.09	0.60	0.29
Sertraline	0.67	0.65	0.63	0.55	0.28	0.18	0.67	0.52
Albuterol	0.88	0.98	0.89	0.67	0.33	0.21	0.53	0.62
Ozempic	850	208	168	148	176	108	84	286
Viagra	70.00	39.00	36.75	44.40	44.00	1.50	28.00	32.50
Insulin	400.00	130.00	94.50	222.00	110.00	4.50	49.00	130.00
Lipitor	0.97	0.39	0.53	0.93	0.55	0.36	0.56	0.85
Atenolol	0.07	0.13	0.21	0.07	0.08	0.06	0.28	0.10
Sumatriptan	10.00	6.50	5.25	4.43	8.25	0.60	7.00	5.20

The market-driven approach in the U.S. contrasts sharply with systems in the European Union (EU) and other developed countries, where governments play a more active role in controlling drug prices. In Europe, national healthcare systems negotiate directly with pharmaceutical companies, using collective bargaining power to set affordable prices that prioritize public health. European governments often implement price controls and encourage the use of generic drugs to maintain lower costs for consumers.

This chapter explores the financial realities of the pharmaceutical industry, comparing U.S. and EU pricing models to illustrate the economic strategies that contribute to the stark price differences. Understanding these pricing mechanisms reveals why Americans pay significantly more for prescription drugs and underscores the impact of market-driven healthcare policies on accessibility and affordability. By examining these factors, we can better understand the financial dynamics shaping the pharmaceutical landscape and the growing demand for reform in U.S. drug pricing practices.

Drug Pricing Strategies: Research and Development (R&D) Costs and Patent Monopolies

One of the most frequently cited reasons for high drug prices is the enormous investment required for research and development (R&D). Pharmaceutical companies argue that the cost of discovering, developing, and testing new drugs is prohibitively high, often exceeding $2.6 billion per drug (DiMasi et al., 2016). These costs include clinical trials, regulatory approval processes, and the extensive time spent researching compounds that may never come to market. Additionally, once a drug is developed, companies must recoup these R&D expenses during the period of market exclusivity, leading to higher initial prices.

Patent monopolies are a critical aspect of drug pricing strategies, allowing pharmaceutical companies to hold exclusive rights to market their drugs for up to 20 years from the date of patent filing (Kesselheim et al., 2018). During this time, no generic competition can legally enter the market, enabling companies to set higher prices without the threat of cheaper alternatives. Patent extensions and strategies like "evergreening"—making minor changes to a drug to extend its patent life—further delay the introduction of generic alternatives, thereby keeping prices high (Hemphill & Sampat, 2012). While patents are essential for incentivizing innovation, the prolonged monopolies in the U.S. contribute significantly to the cost burden on patients.

In contrast, European countries implement stricter controls on patent life extensions and prioritize the early introduction of generics, helping to lower prices once the initial patent expires. These countries also rely on centralized healthcare systems that negotiate directly with pharmaceutical companies to limit the extent of price increases during the patent monopoly period (Morgan et al., 2017).

Price Setting in the U.S. versus the EU and Other Countries

Drug prices in the U.S. are not regulated by the federal government. Pharmaceutical companies are free to set their own prices based on market demand, profitability goals, and competitive considerations. This market-based pricing system contrasts sharply with the approach taken by the European Union (EU) and other developed countries, where governments typically negotiate directly with drug manufacturers to set prices that reflect both the value of the drug and the need to maintain affordability for the population (Wouters et al., 2020).

In the U.S., Medicare, which covers a significant portion of the elderly population, is prohibited by law from negotiating drug prices, leaving the private insurance market as the primary negotiator with pharmaceutical companies (Sarnak et al., 2017). This fragmented system lacks the collective bargaining power seen in countries with single-payer healthcare systems, allowing drug manufacturers to maintain high prices. Insurance companies, in turn, pass these costs onto consumers through higher premiums and out-of-pocket expenses.

European countries, by contrast, have implemented reference pricing, a system in which the government sets drug prices based on the prices of equivalent medications in other countries. Countries like the UK, Germany, and France use cost-effectiveness analyses to determine the value of new drugs and negotiate prices accordingly (Wouters et al., 2020). This system helps keep prices more stable and ensures that life-saving medications are accessible to the population without causing financial hardship.

Market Competition and Its Impact on Pricing

Market competition—or the lack thereof—is a crucial factor in drug pricing, significantly impacting the affordability of medications for consumers. In competitive markets, the introduction of generic drugs typically drives prices down, offering consumers more affordable alternatives to brand-name medications. However, the U.S. pharmaceutical market often lacks this level of competition, especially for newer drugs still protected by patents. Patent protections, designed to allow companies to recoup their research and development costs, also delay the entry of generics, which limits consumer options and enables pharmaceutical companies to retain high prices for extended periods (Kesselheim et al., 2018).

Beyond patents, regulatory hurdles also slow the entry of generics into the U.S. market, prolonging periods of limited competition. Even when generics become eligible for market entry, the use of "pay-for-delay" agreements complicates competition further. In these cases, brand-name manufacturers pay potential generic competitors to delay launching their lower-cost versions, keeping prices artificially high and reducing consumer access to affordable alternatives (Carrier, 2009). These practices contribute to prolonged market dominance for brand-name drugs, often keeping prices elevated for years beyond the original patent period.

In contrast, Europe's pharmaceutical market is more conducive to competition due to regulatory policies that encourage the early introduction of generics. Many EU countries have streamlined approval processes for generics and fewer legal barriers, allowing generic drugs to enter the market more quickly and effectively. Additionally, national health systems within the EU negotiate drug prices directly with pharmaceutical companies, often securing lower costs by leveraging their broad patient bases. These systems not only facilitate faster generic entry but also ensure that prices remain more affordable for consumers (Morgan et al., 2017).

The result is a stark contrast between the U.S. and European markets. In Europe, robust competition through generics and price negotiations contributes to lower prices, while in the U.S., the combination of patent protections, regulatory hurdles, and anti-competitive practices such as pay-for-delay agreements allows brand-name drugs to dominate the market and maintain high prices for longer periods. This disparity highlights the impact of policy and regulatory approaches on drug pricing and underscores the need for reform in the U.S. to foster a more competitive and affordable pharmaceutical market.

Profit Margins: Pharmaceutical Companies in the U.S. versus the EU

The profit margins of pharmaceutical companies in the U.S. are among the highest of any industry, driven in part by the country's unique pricing structure and patent system. On average, U.S. pharmaceutical companies report profit margins of around 15-20%, significantly higher than those of companies in Europe, where margins tend to be closer to 10-15% (Anderson et al., 2019). This disparity is largely due to the fact that U.S. drug prices are higher, giving companies greater leeway to generate profits even after accounting for R&D costs.

In the U.S., companies are not only able to charge more for their products, but they are also able to do so for longer periods due to patent protections and the lack of price regulation. Furthermore, the U.S. system allows pharmaceutical companies to reinvest their profits into marketing and lobbying efforts, further reinforcing their market power (Taylor et al., 2019). In Europe, where governments impose stricter price controls and patent life limitations, profit margins are more modest, and companies are forced to compete on price to secure government contracts.

While the high profitability of U.S. pharmaceutical companies has been defended as necessary to fuel innovation, critics argue that this focus on profit maximization has come at the expense of patient affordability and access to essential medicines (Kesselheim et al., 2018). The EU's focus on balancing innovation with public health priorities presents a stark contrast to the profit-driven nature of the U.S. pharmaceutical market.

The pricing of prescription drugs in the U.S. is a complex issue shaped by patent monopolies, a lack of competition, and an economic system that prioritizes corporate profits over patient affordability. In contrast, European countries have developed systems that balance innovation with the need to provide affordable healthcare, resulting in significantly lower drug prices. By examining the economic forces behind drug pricing, it becomes clear that the U.S. pharmaceutical system is designed to benefit corporate stakeholders, often at the expense of patients who rely on these medications. To address this issue, policymakers must consider reforms that promote competition, limit patent abuses, and introduce price negotiations that reflect the true value of pharmaceutical innovation.

Chapter 4

Government and Price Regulation

The cost of healthcare is a central issue in many countries, but nowhere is the disparity in drug pricing more evident than between the United States and Europe. While U.S. consumers often face high out-of-pocket expenses for medications, European countries have adopted strategies to regulate prices, making life-saving drugs more accessible and affordable. Government intervention plays a pivotal role in this difference, as EU member states negotiate directly with pharmaceutical companies, set reference prices, and leverage the power of centralized healthcare systems to control costs. This chapter delves into the mechanisms behind Europe's approach, exploring how countries like the UK, Germany, and France achieve lower drug prices through structured government policies. By examining these examples, we see the profound impact that regulatory frameworks can have on healthcare affordability, offering insights into the potential benefits and challenges of government-led price controls.

Why Europe Pays Less: The Role of Government Intervention

Pharmaceutical pricing has become a focal point in global health debates, with sharp disparities in drug costs between regions. The United States, known for its high prescription drug prices, contrasts markedly with the European Union (EU), where structured policies help control and regulate these costs to ensure broader affordability. This chapter investigates the key regulatory mechanisms employed by EU countries, highlighting how governmental intervention, strategic price negotiations, and centralized healthcare systems contribute to keeping drug prices lower compared to other regions.

In the EU, healthcare systems are designed to prioritize accessibility and affordability through collective bargaining and stringent pricing policies. Governmental bodies in each country negotiate directly with pharmaceutical companies, setting price ceilings and securing discounted rates for medications. This centralized approach not only allows EU countries to leverage their larger patient populations for better pricing but also introduces a level of cost predictability that benefits both healthcare providers and patients.

The United Kingdom, Germany, and France serve as primary examples of how this model operates. In the UK, the National Health Service (NHS) negotiates drug prices with manufacturers through the National Institute for Health and Care Excellence (NICE), which assesses the cost-effectiveness of new drugs before they are made available to the public. Germany's approach involves a price negotiation process led by the Federal Joint Committee, which evaluates the added benefit of new medications and sets prices accordingly. France's system operates similarly, where the government negotiates directly with pharmaceutical companies based on assessments of therapeutic value and market impact. These policies collectively ensure that prices remain manageable, reducing out-of-pocket expenses for citizens.

By examining these specific policies, this chapter demonstrates how structured government involvement and centralized healthcare systems in the EU help mitigate pharmaceutical costs for European citizens. In contrast to the market-driven model in the U.S., the European approach underscores the effectiveness of direct negotiation and regulatory oversight in maintaining drug affordability, highlighting potential paths for reform in regions where high drug prices pose a significant burden on public health.

The EU's Regulatory Framework for Drug Pricing

The European Union plays a pivotal role in shaping drug prices through policies that prioritize accessibility and affordability. Unlike in the United States, where pharmaceutical companies often set prices with minimal governmental oversight, the EU enforces regulations that place a cap on drug costs. These regulations ensure that drugs, particularly life-saving treatments, remain affordable across member states. The EU achieves this through guidelines that dictate how member countries should approach price negotiations, often involving public health authorities in these discussions to align costs with national healthcare budgets.

This centralized approach benefits EU member countries by standardizing certain aspects of the drug pricing process, giving them collective bargaining power. While individual countries within the EU retain some autonomy, they often adopt similar mechanisms, such as reference pricing systems, which use the prices of specific drugs in other countries as benchmarks. This framework prevents drastic price hikes and makes the pharmaceutical industry accountable for justifying pricing models.

Price Negotiations and Reference Pricing Systems

One of the key strategies used by the EU and its member states to manage drug prices is a combination of price negotiation and reference pricing systems. Reference pricing involves setting a price ceiling for a drug based on its cost in other comparable countries. This approach prevents pharmaceutical companies from charging significantly higher prices in specific countries by establishing a benchmark across borders. For instance, if a drug is sold at a certain price in Germany, other EU countries may use that price as a reference, thus keeping costs consistent and preventing extreme price disparities.

Direct price negotiations with pharmaceutical companies further enhance cost control. In many EU nations, governments engage in negotiations with drug manufacturers to set acceptable prices for medications. In these discussions, companies must provide evidence of the drug's effectiveness and justify its proposed price, often undergoing a detailed review through health technology assessments (HTAs). Countries like France and the UK rely on HTAs to evaluate a drug's clinical and economic value, allowing them to assess its impact on public health and negotiate a price that reflects both the drug's benefits and the financial constraints of the national healthcare system. These assessments examine a drug's efficacy, potential health outcomes, and cost-effectiveness, giving governments leverage to push back against inflated prices.

This combined approach of reference pricing and direct negotiations enables EU countries to maintain a structured framework for regulating pharmaceutical costs. By aligning drug prices across borders and demanding economic justifications for high costs, these strategies create a balanced system where affordability and accessibility are prioritized. This model demonstrates how a regulated pricing system can mitigate the risk of excessive drug costs, offering a potential blueprint for other regions grappling with the challenges of high pharmaceutical prices.

Impact of Centralized Healthcare Systems on Price Control
Centralized healthcare systems are crucial to the EU's success in regulating drug prices effectively. In countries like the UK, where the National Health Service (NHS) provides healthcare to citizens, the government acts as a single, unified buyer for pharmaceuticals. This creates substantial bargaining power, enabling the NHS to negotiate lower prices with pharmaceutical companies. With such consolidated purchasing, the NHS can secure medications at lower prices, ensuring affordable access for UK citizens. Similarly, France's centralized system designates the government as the primary purchaser of pharmaceuticals, establishing strict pricing criteria based on a drug's health impact and cost-effectiveness. This centralized approach allows France to systematically evaluate each drug's value before finalizing its price, preventing unnecessary costs from inflating healthcare expenses.

This centralized model contrasts sharply with systems where multiple private insurers operate, such as in the United States, where price negotiations are fragmented across numerous private entities. In the U.S., private insurers negotiate independently, resulting in inconsistencies and less effective bargaining power. This decentralized negotiation structure weakens the potential to demand lower prices, often leading to higher drug costs for consumers.

Centralized healthcare systems in Europe further streamline the approval and integration of generic drugs, which typically cost significantly less than brand-name versions. By promoting the swift introduction of generics, centralized systems maintain competitive pressure on pharmaceutical companies, which helps keep overall drug prices more affordable. The combination of unified purchasing power and streamlined generic approvals allows centralized systems in the EU to exert substantial influence over pharmaceutical companies, fostering a healthcare environment where cost control and accessibility are achievable goals.

Case Studies: The UK, Germany, and France

Examining individual countries' approaches to drug pricing offers valuable insights into how government policies can influence healthcare costs and access. In Europe, nations such as the UK, Germany, and France have developed distinct, yet similarly effective, models for regulating pharmaceutical prices, each reflecting its unique healthcare system and policy priorities. Through robust negotiation strategies, centralized healthcare structures, and tailored regulatory frameworks, these countries manage to keep drug prices significantly lower than in many other regions. This section delved into each of these models, highlighting how different strategies work within varied healthcare landscapes to control costs, prioritize patient access, and maintain high standards of care. By exploring these examples, we can better understand the practical impact of government-led price regulation and the lessons they offer for global healthcare systems.

- **The United Kingdom**: The UK's NHS has a robust price negotiation system that leverages its role as the sole purchaser of drugs to control costs. Through the National Institute for Health and Care Excellence (NICE), the NHS assesses the cost-effectiveness of new medications before agreeing to cover them. NICE uses quality-adjusted life year (QALY) metrics to decide whether a drug provides sufficient benefit relative to its price, ensuring that only drugs meeting rigorous standards are funded by the NHS.

- **Germany**: Germany's approach includes both free-market elements and government intervention. The country uses a system called AMNOG (Arzneimittelmarkt-Neuordnungsgesetz), which requires pharmaceutical companies to negotiate prices with health insurers within a year of a drug's launch. If the parties fail to agree, an arbitration board sets the price. Germany also uses reference pricing, where drugs are categorized based on similar therapies, establishing a reference price for each group. This approach ensures that new drugs are priced competitively while safeguarding the healthcare system from excessive costs.

- **France**: France's healthcare system is similarly centralized, allowing the government to play a major role in setting drug prices. The Economic Committee for Health Products (CEPS) negotiates prices with pharmaceutical companies, using evaluations by the French National Authority for Health (HAS) to determine each drug's effectiveness. Drugs that provide significant therapeutic benefits are often priced higher, but they are subject to strict pricing reviews and ongoing monitoring. This structured approach ensures that public funds are allocated efficiently, and drugs are priced fairly based on their clinical impact.

Europe's ability to maintain lower drug prices through government intervention and centralized healthcare systems offers valuable insights for countries grappling with high pharmaceutical costs. By employing price negotiations, reference pricing, and centralized purchasing power, the EU effectively balances the need for accessible healthcare with the costs of pharmaceutical innovation. Examples from the UK, Germany, and France demonstrate how a strong regulatory framework and centralized oversight can yield a more sustainable and affordable healthcare system. As other nations, including the United States, seek solutions to soaring drug prices, Europe's model presents a compelling case for the role of government in regulating healthcare costs.

Chapter 5

The Role of Patents and Generic Drugs

In the world of pharmaceuticals, patents hold a powerful sway over drug accessibility and affordability. Intended to reward innovation and encourage investment in new treatments, patents grant drug manufacturers exclusive rights to sell their products, creating a temporary monopoly. Yet, this monopoly often leads to high prices that place essential medicines out of reach for many patients. In contrast, generic drugs—introduced once patents expire—offer a crucial path to affordable healthcare. This chapter explores the dual role of patents as both catalysts for pharmaceutical breakthroughs and barriers to affordable medicine, examining how patent laws, corporate strategies, and the availability of generics shape drug markets in the U.S., Europe, and beyond. Through an analysis of global patent policies and case studies of blockbuster drugs, we gain insight into the complex relationship between intellectual property and public health.

Monopolies in Medicine: Patents and Price Manipulation

Pharmaceutical costs are a global concern, with patent protections at the core of discussions around high drug prices. Patents grant pharmaceutical companies exclusive rights to manufacture and sell their products for a set period, typically 20 years. While these legal monopolies are designed to incentivize innovation by allowing companies to recoup their R&D investments, they often limit access to affordable alternatives. In this chapter, we examine the contrasting approaches to patent protections in the U.S. and Europe, highlighting how these policies impact drug costs and access to life-saving treatments.

The U.S. patent system is particularly favorable to pharmaceutical companies, with strong protections that often enable them to retain exclusivity beyond the initial patent term. Through practices like "evergreening," companies make minor modifications to existing drugs to extend patent protections, delaying the introduction of lower-cost generics. This strategy allows high-revenue drugs to dominate the market for extended periods, keeping prices elevated and limiting affordable options for consumers. Case studies of drugs like insulin and popular cancer treatments reveal how patent extensions can lead to prolonged periods of high costs, even as patients face significant financial strain.

In contrast, Europe takes a more balanced approach to patent protections, implementing stricter regulations around patent extensions and encouraging the faster entry of generic drugs. Many European countries limit evergreening and provide incentives for companies to introduce generics once the initial patent expires. This regulatory framework promotes competition and helps to drive down prices more quickly than in the U.S., making critical drugs more affordable. Countries like Germany and France rely on centralized health agencies to set price limits on drugs, allowing the government to negotiate and impose cost restrictions that are difficult to enforce in a fragmented, market-driven system like the U.S.

Globally, countries adopt various strategies to balance innovation with affordable healthcare. Nations with robust generic drug markets, such as India and Brazil, prioritize accessibility by fast-tracking generic approvals, often in defiance of extended patent protections. These countries have cultivated thriving generic industries, which provide affordable alternatives to brand-name drugs and supply much-needed medications to low- and middle-income populations.

By comparing the patent policies and generic markets across the U.S., Europe, and other regions, this chapter illustrates the impact of patent protections on drug prices and accessibility. Understanding these differences highlights the challenges in balancing innovation incentives with the need for affordable healthcare and underscores potential pathways to reform that prioritize patient access without stifling pharmaceutical innovation.

Patents and Intellectual Property: A Comparison Between the U.S. and Europe

The United States and Europe approach patent protections for pharmaceuticals differently, with significant implications for drug affordability and accessibility. In the U.S., pharmaceutical companies generally receive a 20-year patent for new drugs, but extensions are frequently granted through a practice known as "evergreening." Evergreening allows companies to maintain exclusivity by making minor modifications to an existing drug—such as altering dosage forms or formulations—which extends the patent life and delays the entry of lower-cost generics into the market (Abbott & Vernon, 2007). This practice contributes to the persistence of high drug prices in the U.S., as brand-name drugs retain their market dominance well beyond the original patent expiration.

In contrast, European policies are structured to limit such patent extensions and prioritize faster access to affordable generics. The European Union uses mechanisms like the Supplementary Protection Certificate (SPC), which provides a more controlled extension period—usually up to five years—specifically to offset the time required for regulatory approval. However, this extension is capped, ensuring that generics can enter the market relatively soon after the patent expires, compared to the U.S. (European Commission, 2022). This system aligns with Europe's broader emphasis on public health accessibility, as it balances the need for rewarding innovation with a commitment to affordability and accessibility.

The European approach to limiting patent extensions reflects a regulatory philosophy that prioritizes public health over extended market exclusivity, underscoring a stark difference from the U.S. model. By limiting the duration of exclusivity, European countries promote competition and reduce drug prices more effectively than the U.S., where longer patent protections often restrict market competition. This divergence in patent policies highlights the tension between fostering pharmaceutical innovation and ensuring affordable access to medications, illuminating the complex interplay between intellectual property laws and public health priorities across different regulatory landscapes (Gleeson et al., 2019).

These differences in patent handling between the U.S. and Europe underscore the global challenge of balancing incentives for pharmaceutical innovation with the urgent need for affordable healthcare. While U.S. policies favor extended exclusivity, Europe's more restrictive approach aims to make medicines accessible sooner, promoting a model where patient access is a primary concern. This comparative analysis demonstrates that regulatory policies can profoundly shape drug pricing and availability, with each system offering insights for potential reforms that consider both innovation and patient welfare.

Blockbuster Drugs: How Patents Keep Prices High

The influence of patents on drug pricing is especially evident with blockbuster drugs that generate substantial revenue. AbbVie's Humira, a treatment for autoimmune conditions, exemplifies how extended patent protection strategies can sustain high prices. Through a series of secondary patents on Humira's formulations and delivery methods, AbbVie effectively blocked generic competition in the U.S. long after the original patent expired. This approach allowed the company to continue charging as much as $60,000 annually per patient, while European markets, governed by stricter patent regulations, saw affordable biosimilar versions enter sooner, resulting in reduced prices for European patients (Feldman, 2018; Staton, 2021).

Similar tactics are widespread in the insulin market, where manufacturers repeatedly modify existing formulas and delivery devices to renew patents, hindering the introduction of affordable biosimilar alternatives. These extended monopolies keep costs high for patients who rely on life-saving insulin, sparking ethical concerns around accessibility. Many argue that such practices place profits over patient welfare, as high prices for essential medications force patients to make difficult financial choices or go without necessary treatments (Thomas, Capstick, & Kesselheim, 2016).

This trend has increasingly attracted public and policy scrutiny. Patients, healthcare providers, and advocates are calling for reforms to curb these patent extension tactics, arguing that prolonged monopolies on critical drugs run counter to public health interests. The cases of Humira and insulin illustrate the broader ethical dilemma: how to balance the protection of pharmaceutical innovation with the need for affordable access to life-saving treatments. As scrutiny intensifies, policymakers are exploring solutions that would limit these practices, aiming to foster a pharmaceutical market where critical medications remain within reach for those who need them most.

Generic Drug Availability and the U.S. Market's Slow Adoption
Despite the prevalence of generics in the U.S., their introduction often faces significant delays compared to Europe. Brand-name pharmaceutical companies in the U.S. commonly employ legal tactics to postpone generic competition, including "pay-for-delay" agreements. In these arrangements, brand-name manufacturers compensate generic companies to delay the release of their lower-cost versions, extending the brand's market exclusivity and keeping prices high for an extended period (Carrier, 2009). These practices have far-reaching implications for consumers and healthcare systems, as they prevent competition and restrict access to affordable medications.

In contrast, European countries have implemented streamlined approval processes that encourage the rapid entry of generics soon after patent expiration. Without the obstacles common in the U.S., European generics reach the market faster, often leading to significant reductions in drug costs. Studies have shown that the increased availability of generics in Europe drives down drug prices, providing cost-saving benefits for both patients and national healthcare systems (Dylst, Vulto, & Simoens, 2013).

These contrasting approaches illustrate how policy frameworks influence access to affordable medications. Europe's regulatory environment, which promotes quicker generic approval and discourages anti-competitive practices, prioritizes cost-effective alternatives. This focus not only benefits consumers but also reduces the financial strain on healthcare budgets. The U.S., by allowing extended patent strategies and delayed generics, faces persistent challenges with high drug prices, underscoring the potential impact of policy reforms that facilitate access to affordable generics.

Global Comparison of Generic Drug Markets and Competition
Globally, variations in generic drug availability underscore the importance of balanced patent policies. Countries like India, which has adopted shorter patent exclusivity periods, have established robust generic industries, providing affordable medication to millions worldwide (Chaudhuri, Goldberg, & Jia, 2006). Known as the "pharmacy of the developing world," India supplies affordable generics to countries that cannot afford high-priced brand-name drugs, illustrating the benefits of reduced patent restrictions.

In contrast, countries with stricter patent protections, including the United States, experience higher drug costs due to limited generic competition. Comparative studies show that countries with streamlined access to generics enjoy greater competition and reduced prices, which contributes to better public health outcomes (Watal, 2000). By examining these international examples, it becomes evident that patent policies profoundly influence both the affordability of healthcare and access to life-saving treatments.

Patents and intellectual property rights profoundly impact the accessibility and pricing of pharmaceuticals. While patents drive innovation, they also create monopolies that can inflate drug prices, restricting access to essential medications. The U.S. patent system allows extensive protection, contributing to higher costs and slower generic adoption compared to Europe. As other countries pursue solutions to escalating healthcare costs, the balance between encouraging innovation and ensuring public access to affordable drugs remains a key challenge for policymakers.

Chapter 6

Lobbying and Political Influence

The influence of pharmaceutical companies over American politics has shaped the landscape of healthcare policy in profound ways. With billions of dollars spent each year on lobbying and campaign contributions, Big Pharma has positioned itself as one of the most powerful interest groups in Washington. This influence is not merely about access; it extends to shaping policy, protecting profit margins, and blocking reforms that could lower drug prices for consumers. As a result, efforts to make medications more affordable often face fierce opposition, stalling or diluting legislative progress. In this chapter, we explore the extensive lobbying efforts of the pharmaceutical industry, its impact on policy, and the consequences for American patients, examining how Big Pharma's political power has perpetuated a healthcare system that prioritizes profits over public health.

Big Pharma's Grip on American Politics

The pharmaceutical industry wields substantial influence over policy in the United States, shaping legislation, regulation, and public perception through extensive lobbying and political contributions. Known collectively as "Big Pharma," these corporations spend billions of dollars annually to shape drug-related policies, often placing profit motives above public interest. This chapter explores the scale of pharmaceutical lobbying, its impact on drug pricing and healthcare policy, and contrasts this environment with Europe, where lobbying efforts are less pervasive and more regulated.

In the U.S., pharmaceutical companies rank among the highest-spending industries on lobbying activities, aiming to influence everything from drug pricing and patent laws to regulatory oversight and healthcare access. Political contributions to key policymakers and lobbying of regulatory agencies often create a favorable environment for industry priorities, which can include extended patent protections, limited price controls, and lax restrictions on marketing. By contributing to political campaigns and working directly with legislators, Big Pharma has effectively shaped a policy landscape that frequently prioritizes corporate profits over affordability and accessibility for consumers.

Comparatively, European countries maintain stricter regulations on lobbying and have developed healthcare systems where governments play a more active role in drug price negotiations and regulation. With national health systems as primary purchasers of medications, European governments maintain more bargaining power and are less susceptible to lobbying pressures. Consequently, drug prices in Europe are generally lower, and the influence of pharmaceutical companies on policy is significantly curtailed.

Case studies highlight the influence of pharmaceutical lobbying on American healthcare. For instance, efforts to limit Medicare's ability to negotiate drug prices, largely backed by industry-funded lobbying, have kept U.S. drug costs among the highest in the world. Additionally, lobbying efforts supporting extended patent protections and practices like "evergreening" have preserved market exclusivity for high-revenue drugs, restricting affordable generics.

These differences in regulatory environments illustrate how pharmaceutical lobbying shapes the U.S. healthcare system, often resulting in high costs and limited access to affordable treatments. By comparing the U.S. to Europe, this chapter underscores the profound impact of industry influence on healthcare policy and highlights the potential for policy reforms that limit lobbying's role in favor of prioritizing patient access and public health.

Pharmaceutical Industry Lobbying Efforts in the U.S.

The pharmaceutical industry ranks as one of the most powerful lobbying forces in the United States, dedicating significant resources to shaping policy through Congress, regulatory agencies, and public opinion (OpenSecrets, 2022). Pharmaceutical companies collectively spend over $300 million annually on lobbying efforts, with major corporations like Pfizer, Johnson & Johnson, and Merck leading the charge (Proctor, 2021). These efforts primarily focus on protecting patent exclusivity, opposing price regulation, and advocating for favorable tax and intellectual property policies.

Industry associations like the Pharmaceutical Research and Manufacturers of America (PhRMA) play a critical role in amplifying these lobbying activities. PhRMA, for instance, invests millions to promote policies that align with the industry's interests, maintaining close relationships with influential policymakers. The association's access to key decision-makers is bolstered by the presence of former government officials who take on strategic roles within pharmaceutical companies or industry organizations, creating a "revolving door" that often aligns industry priorities with legislative outcomes (Carpenter, 2014).

These extensive lobbying efforts allow Big Pharma to shape policy discussions to favor corporate objectives, often prioritizing profit protection over consumer affordability and access. For example, lobbying campaigns by pharmaceutical companies have repeatedly challenged proposals to limit drug prices or expand Medicare's negotiating power. Similarly, advocacy to extend patent protections through practices like "evergreening" has helped pharmaceutical companies preserve exclusivity for profitable drugs, often delaying the availability of affordable generics.

The scale and influence of pharmaceutical lobbying reveal a complex interplay between industry interests and public policy, underscoring the industry's capacity to protect its economic priorities in ways that can disadvantage consumers. By securing favorable policies, often through direct access to lawmakers and regulatory bodies, Big Pharma has sustained a healthcare landscape where high drug prices are prevalent, underscoring the need for regulatory reforms that prioritize consumer welfare over corporate interests.

Political Influence: How Campaign Donations and Lobbying Affect Policy

Campaign donations are a potent strategy Big Pharma uses to secure favorable policies, contributing to both Democratic and Republican campaigns to ensure bipartisan support for its objectives (Sachs, 2021). These contributions often surge during legislative cycles that could impact drug pricing or patent protections, especially when discussions involve patent exclusivity periods or potential pricing regulations (Taylor & Gomez, 2019). By supporting key lawmakers across the political spectrum, pharmaceutical companies effectively build alliances that influence policy outcomes to favor their financial interests.

The industry's influence is further bolstered by the "revolving door" phenomenon, where individuals frequently move between roles in government and the pharmaceutical sector. Former regulatory officials, after leaving their government positions, often take up strategic roles within pharmaceutical companies, leveraging their insider knowledge and established networks to shape policy and regulatory decisions from within the industry (Ornstein & Weber, 2018). This exchange of personnel facilitates relationships that strengthen Big Pharma's access to policymakers, creating a feedback loop that perpetuates industry-friendly policies.

The combined effects of campaign donations and the revolving door result in regulatory and legislative environments that frequently favor Big Pharma's priorities, often at the expense of competition and consumer affordability. These influences have contributed to policies that restrict generic drug approvals, extend patent exclusivity through practices like "evergreening," and protect high drug prices. This system burdens both consumers, who face high out-of-pocket costs, and taxpayers, who fund government healthcare programs affected by these inflated prices. Together, campaign donations and the revolving door highlight how pharmaceutical industry practices shape U.S. drug policy, underscoring the need for reforms that prioritize public health and affordability over corporate profit.

Case Studies of Legislation Shaped by Pharmaceutical Interests
To understand Big Pharma's influence, consider the following legislative cases shaped by lobbying and campaign contributions:

- Medicare Prescription Drug, Improvement, and Modernization Act of 2003: This law, which created Medicare Part D, prohibits Medicare from negotiating drug prices, leading to higher costs for taxpayers. Industry lobbying heavily influenced this provision, allowing pharmaceutical companies to set high prices for Medicare-covered drugs without government intervention (Geyman, 2015).

- Biologics Price Competition and Innovation Act of 2009: This legislation established an approval pathway for biosimilars (generic versions of biologic drugs). However, industry lobbying led to a 12-year exclusivity period for biologics, limiting market competition and keeping prices high for medications used in critical treatments (Kesselheim et al., 2011).

- The 21st Century Cures Act (2016): Heavily backed by Big Pharma, this act streamlined drug approvals, purportedly to enhance patient access, but critics argue it lowered safety standards. The law allowed products to enter the market more quickly, often without rigorous oversight, benefiting manufacturers (Zuckerman & Browne, 2017).

These cases illustrate how pharmaceutical lobbying shapes legislation, often prioritizing profit over public welfare. Through significant financial contributions and strategic partnerships, pharmaceutical companies exert influence over lawmakers, steering policy decisions that favor corporate interests rather than the needs of patients. This dynamic creates an environment where essential reforms aimed at lowering drug prices and improving access to medications are consistently undermined, perpetuating a system that prioritizes revenue generation over the health and well-being of the public.

Comparison to the Regulatory Environment in Europe and Other Countries

Unlike in the U.S., where lobbying heavily influences drug policy, Europe maintains stricter lobbying restrictions and prioritizes public health over corporate profit. Many European countries regulate drug prices through centralized healthcare systems that negotiate prices directly with manufacturers, limiting pharmaceutical lobbying influence (Kanavos et al., 2011).

For instance, in the UK, corporate political donations are highly regulated, reducing Big Pharma's influence on policy. In addition, European governments use independent health technology assessments (HTAs) to evaluate drug cost-effectiveness, preventing lobbying from swaying policy (Cohen et al., 2010). This contrast highlights how limitations on lobbying can improve healthcare affordability and outcomes.

The pharmaceutical industry's substantial investment in lobbying and political contributions grants it significant influence over U.S. healthcare policy, often resulting in legislation that favors corporate profits over public affordability and access. Through lobbying, campaign donations, and the revolving door, Big Pharma shapes drug pricing, patent laws, and regulatory processes. By comparison, Europe's restricted lobbying practices, centralized healthcare systems, and independent policy assessments promote a more consumer-friendly healthcare landscape. Addressing the influence of Big Pharma in the U.S. is essential for achieving fairer healthcare policies that prioritize public health.

Chapter 7

Direct-to-Consumer Advertising

In the world of modern healthcare, advertising has become as familiar as the prescriptions it promotes. Direct-to-consumer (DTC) advertising, where pharmaceutical companies market prescription drugs directly to the public, is unique to the United States and New Zealand, standing out as an anomaly in global healthcare. Supporters argue that DTC advertising empowers patients by informing them of treatment options, but critics see it as a powerful tool that promotes a culture of over-medication, inflates drug prices, and drives healthcare costs upward. With ads that encourage viewers to "ask your doctor" about the latest brand-name drug, DTC advertising transforms the doctor-patient relationship, placing pharmaceutical companies at the heart of medical decisions. This chapter explores the far-reaching impacts of DTC advertising on drug costs, patient behavior, and healthcare systems, examining how the promise of empowerment may actually be selling sickness.

Selling Sickness: The Role of Drug Advertising in America

Direct-to-consumer (DTC) advertising, a practice where pharmaceutical companies market prescription drugs directly to the public, is a uniquely American phenomenon, with the United States and New Zealand being the only countries that permit it. This strategy allows drug companies to reach patients through television, online platforms, and print media, profoundly shaping consumer perceptions, drug demand, and the overall healthcare system. While proponents argue that DTC advertising educates patients about treatment options, critics suggest it contributes to escalating drug prices, encourages over-prescription, and fosters a culture where medical solutions are equated primarily with pharmaceuticals.

DTC advertising has a notable impact on drug prices. High marketing expenses drive up costs, which pharmaceutical companies often pass on to consumers. To maintain a competitive edge, companies invest heavily in advertising campaigns for their newest, often higher-priced drugs, positioning these medications as first-line solutions, regardless of whether less expensive alternatives might be available. This practice reinforces brand loyalty and demand for patented drugs, which limits competition and can delay the adoption of more affordable generic options.

The psychological impact of DTC advertising on patients is significant. By targeting consumers directly, pharmaceutical companies can create awareness but also anxiety, sometimes encouraging patients to seek prescriptions for drugs they may not need. The commercials often employ persuasive messaging that suggests medication is a quick solution, influencing patients to request specific drugs from their doctors. This approach can shift the doctor-patient dynamic, pressuring healthcare providers to prescribe advertised medications, even when they might not be the most appropriate choice. Such trends contribute to a healthcare culture where medication is often prioritized over non-drug treatments or lifestyle changes.

In contrast, most other countries enforce strict advertising restrictions on prescription medications to prioritize public health and reduce healthcare costs. European countries, for example, prohibit DTC advertising, allowing only factual drug information to be shared through regulated channels, which helps prevent the over-medicalization of health issues. By limiting advertising, these countries foster a healthcare environment where treatment decisions are primarily driven by medical expertise rather than consumer demand, contributing to more judicious prescribing practices and potentially lower drug costs.

This chapter explores the multifaceted impacts of DTC advertising on the U.S. healthcare system, comparing it with international approaches that emphasize public health safeguards. The examination reveals how unrestricted advertising can drive up drug prices and influence patient behavior, highlighting the need for policies that balance consumer education with the protection of public health.

How Pharmaceutical Advertising Affects Drug Prices

Direct-to-consumer (DTC) advertising represents a substantial financial commitment for pharmaceutical companies, costing billions annually. Proponents within the industry argue that this investment is essential for educating consumers on treatment options, empowering them to make informed decisions about their health. However, critics contend that these advertising expenses are ultimately passed on to patients through higher drug prices, contributing significantly to the escalating cost of healthcare (Mintzes, 2012).

Pharmaceutical companies incorporate these marketing expenses directly into the pricing of their medications. For instance, blockbuster drugs like Humira and Lipitor experienced significant price hikes as companies funneled massive sums into their advertising budgets (Schwartz & Woloshin, 2019). As a result, patients bear the cost of these marketing campaigns, often paying considerably more for medications promoted in DTC ads compared to less-advertised, lower-cost alternatives.

A major focus of DTC advertising is on brand-name drugs, encouraging consumers to request these specific medications from their healthcare providers. This approach tends to inflate healthcare costs, as patients often favor branded options over equally effective but less expensive generics. By promoting demand for the newest, often most expensive drugs, DTC advertising fosters a cycle wherein companies set high prices to cover their advertising investments. This strategy not only keeps prices elevated but often leads to additional price increases as the demand for these drugs continues to grow (Rosenthal et al., 2016).

Beyond direct cost impacts, DTC advertising influences patient behavior and prescription practices, contributing to what some view as unnecessary medicalization. By positioning medications as a primary solution for a wide array of health concerns, DTC ads drive demand not only for necessary treatments but also for drugs that may have equally effective, lower-cost alternatives. The economic implications of this approach reverberate throughout the healthcare system, contributing to inflated drug prices, increased insurance premiums, and higher out-of-pocket expenses for patients.

The U.S. and New Zealand: The Only Two Countries Where DTC Advertising is Legal

The United States and New Zealand are the only two countries that permit direct-to-consumer (DTC) advertising of pharmaceuticals, a policy choice that prompts debate about its impact on public health and the overall cost of healthcare. In the U.S., DTC advertisements are regulated by the Food and Drug Administration (FDA), which requires pharmaceutical companies to disclose potential risks and side effects to consumers. However, critics argue that these disclosures are often presented in a way that downplays risks, emphasizing positive aspects through upbeat visuals, music, and testimonials, which can lead consumers to perceive drugs as safer or more effective than they are (Donohue, Cevasco, & Rosenthal, 2007).

New Zealand's approach differs slightly, as the country enforces stricter content guidelines on DTC advertising. Yet, despite these additional safeguards, studies show that DTC ads still lead to increased consumer demand for the advertised drugs. Patients frequently request these medications from healthcare providers, even when there are equally effective, more affordable options available (Toop et al., 2003). This trend puts additional strain on healthcare providers, who must navigate patient expectations while making responsible, cost-effective treatment recommendations.

In both countries, the prevalence of DTC advertising raises critical questions about the role of pharmaceutical marketing in shaping consumer healthcare choices. Proponents argue that DTC advertising enhances public awareness, informing consumers about potential treatment options. However, detractors highlight that DTC advertising can lead to overprescription and misaligned treatment decisions, prioritizing brand-name drugs over more appropriate or cost-effective treatments.

This section probed into how the United States and New Zealand justify permitting DTC pharmaceutical advertising, examining the regulatory frameworks they have in place and the challenges they face in balancing public health interests with the powerful influence of drug marketing on consumer choices.

Psychological Impacts of Advertising on Drug Consumption and Healthcare Costs

Pharmaceutical advertising significantly shapes patient behavior, fostering a demand-driven approach to healthcare that can lead to over-diagnosis and over-treatment. Studies indicate that direct-to-consumer (DTC) advertising prompts patients to seek specific drugs they've seen in ads, often without a clear clinical need, thereby increasing healthcare costs and contributing to the "selling sickness" phenomenon. This concept describes how advertising encourages consumers to interpret everyday health variations as needing medical intervention, driving unnecessary consumption and inflating overall healthcare expenditures (Frosch, Krueger, Hornik, Cronholm, & Barg, 2007).

The psychological effects of DTC advertising are profound, often creating heightened health anxiety among consumers. By portraying minor symptoms as indicators of serious conditions, pharmaceutical ads can amplify concerns, leading patients to request tests, treatments, or medications that might be unnecessary. This not only strains healthcare providers but also leads to a healthcare culture that equates health solutions with pharmaceuticals, sidelining alternative approaches and preventive care. Such advertising-driven behavior places a burden on healthcare systems as doctor visits and prescription requests surge (Moynihan, Heath, & Henry, 2002).

Advertising also influences perceptions around drug quality, often positioning branded medications as superior to generics. Patients, exposed to sophisticated messaging, may develop a bias favoring brand-name drugs, even when generics provide equivalent efficacy at much lower costs. This misconception further drives up healthcare costs as patients and providers prioritize higher-priced options over cost-effective generics, reinforcing a consumer preference that aligns more with advertising influence than clinical evidence (Mintzes, 2012).

This section delves into how DTC advertising leverages psychological triggers to shape patient behavior, leading to higher healthcare expenditures. By examining these dynamics, we can better understand the need for policies that balance consumer awareness with the imperative to prevent unnecessary medicalization and promote informed, cost-effective healthcare choices.

Advertising Bans and Restrictions in the EU and Other Countries

Outside the United States and New Zealand, most countries prohibit or strictly regulate DTC pharmaceutical advertising, prioritizing public health over consumer marketing. In the European Union, direct advertising of prescription drugs to the public is banned, with the goal of preventing undue influence on patients and doctors (Hemminki, 2010). Instead, European pharmaceutical companies focus on educating healthcare providers, who then guide patients in making informed decisions based on clinical evidence rather than promotional messages.

Countries like Canada and Australia allow only limited advertising, with significant restrictions on content to ensure that advertisements do not encourage unnecessary prescriptions. This regulatory environment reflects a public health-oriented approach, where the focus is on protecting consumers from commercial influences that could lead to inappropriate drug use (Lexchin & Mintzes, 2002). This section examines how these international approaches contrast with the U.S. model, highlighting the benefits and challenges of restricting pharmaceutical advertising to promote a more sustainable healthcare system.

DTC advertising in the U.S. and New Zealand creates a unique healthcare landscape where pharmaceutical companies play a direct role in shaping consumer perceptions and driving drug demand. While proponents argue that DTC advertising empowers patients with information, the practice also inflates drug prices, promotes brand-name medications over generics, and can lead to over-prescription and increased healthcare costs. By examining the restrictions placed on pharmaceutical advertising in the EU and other countries, we gain insight into alternative regulatory models that prioritize public health. Limiting DTC advertising could help control drug prices and reduce the burden of unnecessary medication, creating a more balanced and patient-centered healthcare system.

Chapter 8

The Impact on Patients and Healthcare Systems

The rising cost of prescription drugs in the United States has profound and far-reaching effects, impacting not only individual patients but the healthcare system as a whole. As prices for essential medications climb, millions of Americans face difficult choices: rationing their prescriptions, delaying treatment, or foregoing it altogether. These decisions have serious health consequences, leading to preventable complications, hospitalizations, and even premature death. Beyond the individual impact, high drug prices also strain the broader healthcare system, increasing insurance premiums, driving up healthcare costs, and burdening government programs like Medicare and Medicaid. In this chapter, we examine the human toll of high drug prices, the economic burden on the healthcare system, and compare these challenges with healthcare models in other countries, exploring the devastating consequences of an unsustainable drug pricing system and the urgent need for reform.

The Human Cost: How High Prices Affect Patients

The rising cost of prescription drugs in the United States transcends mere financial strain; it is a deeply personal and societal issue, affecting the health and lives of countless individuals. For many Americans, high drug prices present heartbreaking choices: should they cut back on essentials like groceries, delay paying utility bills, or forego needed medications altogether? For patients with chronic or life-threatening conditions, these impossible decisions can mean the difference between life and death. The human impact of unaffordable medications is profound, with high prices preventing individuals from accessing life-saving treatments and worsening health disparities across the nation.

Beyond individual hardship, the economic burden of escalating drug costs reverberates throughout the U.S. healthcare system. High prescription prices drive up insurance premiums, out-of-pocket expenses, and overall healthcare costs, placing an enormous strain on the healthcare system and increasing national healthcare expenditures. This, in turn, affects employers, taxpayers, and the government, as resources are stretched to cover rising expenses linked to inflated drug prices.

In contrast, the European Union offers a valuable comparison. Through stringent price controls and government-led negotiations, EU countries have created a system that prioritizes affordability and accessibility. Regulated drug prices allow European healthcare systems to provide essential medications to patients without excessive financial barriers, contributing to better health outcomes and a more sustainable healthcare model. This approach illustrates how regulatory policies can safeguard public health by reducing cost burdens and ensuring that medications remain within reach for all.

This chapter highlights real stories of American patients affected by high drug costs, illustrating the devastating personal toll of unaffordable prescriptions. It also examines the broader economic impact on the U.S. healthcare system, the comparative advantages of EU drug pricing policies, and how gaps in insurance coverage exacerbate drug affordability challenges. By exploring these facets, we gain a comprehensive view of the prescription drug crisis in the U.S. and the urgent need for reforms that prioritize both economic sustainability and equitable healthcare access.

Stories of Patients Impacted by High Drug Prices in the U.S.

The effects of high drug prices in the United States are most profoundly experienced by individuals who depend on life-saving medications for chronic conditions like diabetes, cancer, or autoimmune diseases. For these patients, the financial challenge of affording medications is a relentless struggle. Insulin, for example—a medication essential for millions of Americans with diabetes—has seen an alarming rise in price over the past few decades. As a result, many patients are forced to ration doses or skip them entirely, which significantly jeopardizes their health and increases the risk of complications (Greene & Riggs, 2019).

Take Sarah's story: a young woman living with type 1 diabetes, she faces monthly insulin costs exceeding $400, even with insurance. This financial burden adds tremendous stress as she tries to balance these expenses alongside rent and other living costs. For patients like James, who relies on biologic medications to manage his rheumatoid arthritis, the cost of treatment can reach an overwhelming $5,000 per month without sufficient insurance coverage. These staggering expenses force difficult choices, often compelling patients to sacrifice basic necessities to afford their medications.

Stories like Sarah's and James's are far from isolated. Across the U.S., countless individuals are forced into impossible decisions between obtaining critical medications and covering essential living expenses. The prevalence of such situations underscores the life-altering impact of high drug prices, highlighting the urgent need for policy interventions that ensure access to affordable, life-saving medications for all.

The Economic Burden of Prescriptions on the American Healthcare System

The high cost of medications extends beyond individual patients, imposing a significant strain on the U.S. healthcare system as a whole. In 2022, Americans spent an estimated $600 billion on prescription drugs, positioning pharmaceuticals as one of the largest drivers of healthcare spending (IQVIA, 2023). This financial impact permeates through hospitals, insurers, and government programs like Medicare and Medicaid, resulting in higher premiums and increased healthcare costs that are ultimately absorbed by patients and taxpayers (Dieguez et al., 2020).

Medicare, which provides essential coverage to millions of elderly and disabled Americans, faces a unique disadvantage: it is legally barred from negotiating drug prices directly with pharmaceutical companies. This restriction contributes to the inflated costs of medications, as Medicare must pay the listed prices set by manufacturers, particularly for brand-name drugs, which are often among the most expensive. Consequently, this lack of price negotiation not only escalates federal spending but also leads to higher premiums for Medicare enrollees, further burdening both beneficiaries and the federal budget (Huang & Catlin, 2021).

Hospitals, too, are impacted by high drug prices, especially when they cover the cost of costly medications for uninsured or underinsured patients. This financial strain can deplete hospital resources, reducing their ability to allocate funds toward other critical services and potentially affecting the quality of care they provide.

This section examines the widespread economic toll of high drug prices, analyzing the ripple effects on private insurers, government budgets, and ultimately, American taxpayers. The impact reverberates across the healthcare system, illustrating how high drug prices exacerbate healthcare costs and limit financial sustainability within public and private health services alike.

Comparison with the EU: How Lower Prices Improve Healthcare Outcomes

While high drug prices continue to burden the U.S. healthcare system, the European Union provides a contrasting model where regulated drug prices contribute to better healthcare outcomes and greater affordability. Through government-led price negotiations and reference pricing systems, EU countries are able to cap costs and ensure that essential medications remain accessible to the public. For example, in Germany and the UK, centralized healthcare systems negotiate drug prices directly with manufacturers, enabling them to secure more affordable prices for patients (Kanavos et al., 2011).

Lower drug prices in the EU also lead to better health outcomes, as patients are more likely to adhere to prescribed treatments without the financial stress often experienced in the U.S. In countries like France, where essential medications are fully or partially covered by the government, patients have better access to treatments and are less likely to skip medications due to cost (Dylst et al., 2013). This section discusses the implications of the EU model, examining how price regulations not only relieve patients of the financial burden but also support broader public health goals by reducing preventable hospitalizations and chronic health complications. The EU's approach offers insight into the benefits of price regulation as a means to improve healthcare outcomes and mitigate economic strain.

Insurance Coverage Gaps and Their Effects on Drug Affordability

The Affordable Care Act (ACA), while expanding healthcare access for millions of Americans, fell short in addressing the rising costs of insurance premiums for individuals and businesses alike. Though the ACA aimed to make insurance more affordable, it did not directly control premium prices. Instead, it relied on mandates and subsidies to offset costs for lower-income individuals, without adequately addressing the underlying factors driving premiums upward. As a result, the cost burden on individuals and companies has continued to grow, often making insurance prohibitively expensive.

For companies, especially small and mid-sized businesses, the ACA presented new challenges. Employers with 50 or more full-time employees were required to provide health insurance or face penalties, yet the rising premiums created a substantial financial strain, especially as healthcare costs increased faster than inflation. Companies offering insurance saw their costs climb, often resulting in reduced benefits, higher deductibles, and cost-sharing measures that shifted a greater portion of the financial burden onto employees.

For individuals purchasing insurance on the ACA marketplace, the story is similar. Premiums have steadily risen, with many middle-income families ineligible for subsidies facing significant out-of-pocket costs. The ACA's income-based subsidies provide some relief, but they do not extend far enough to protect a large segment of consumers from high premiums and deductibles. In practice, these rising costs have left individuals and businesses shouldering more of the financial load, limiting the ACA's effectiveness in truly making healthcare affordable.

This failure to address the drivers of premium inflation underscores a critical gap in the ACA's framework. While the law successfully expanded coverage, the ongoing rise in insurance costs for both individuals and companies has made it clear that more comprehensive reform is needed to tackle the root causes of high healthcare expenses.

The human cost of high drug prices in the United States extends far beyond dollars and cents, affecting patients' well-being, healthcare access, and overall quality of life. Personal stories highlight the daily struggles faced by those who cannot afford their prescribed medications, while the economic burden on the healthcare system underscores the far-reaching impact of high pharmaceutical costs. By contrasting the U.S. system with Europe, where price controls lead to improved healthcare outcomes, it becomes evident that lower drug prices benefit both patients and healthcare infrastructures. Finally, addressing the gaps in insurance coverage is essential for creating a more equitable healthcare environment, ensuring that all patients have access to the medications they need. Reducing the economic and human toll of high drug prices remains a pressing issue for patients, policymakers, and the future of American healthcare.

Chapter 9

Alternatives to the American System

While Americans grapple with high drug prices, many other countries have established systems to keep medications affordable and accessible. Nations like Canada, Germany, and Japan provide valuable models for regulating drug costs through government-led negotiations, price caps, and policies that prioritize public health. These approaches ensure that essential medicines remain within reach for all citizens without compromising the profitability necessary for innovation. In this chapter, we explore these international models, detailing how government intervention, centralized healthcare systems, and price transparency create a more balanced approach to drug pricing. By examining these alternatives, we gain insight into what could be adapted for the U.S., offering a potential path toward a sustainable and equitable healthcare system.

Lessons from Abroad: How Other Countries Keep Prices Low

While the United States struggles with high drug prices and limited access to affordable medications, other countries have implemented effective strategies to keep pharmaceutical costs manageable and accessible for their citizens. Countries such as Canada, Australia, and Japan have developed healthcare systems that prioritize affordability, employing government-led negotiations, transparent pricing practices, and policy frameworks that emphasize public welfare over corporate profit. These international models offer valuable insights into potential reforms for the U.S. pharmaceutical landscape, showcasing practical solutions that align economic sustainability with patient access.

In Canada, the Patented Medicine Prices Review Board (PMPRB) plays a central role in regulating drug prices. Through direct negotiations with pharmaceutical companies, the PMPRB sets maximum prices for medications based on factors such as therapeutic value, price comparisons with other countries, and the average income levels of Canadians. This approach keeps prices consistently affordable, allowing citizens access to essential medications without excessive financial strain.

Australia's Pharmaceutical Benefits Scheme (PBS) takes a similar approach, leveraging the power of a centralized healthcare system to negotiate favorable drug prices. Through the PBS, the Australian government covers the cost of essential medications, setting standardized prices and determining reimbursement rates based on cost-effectiveness analyses. By prioritizing patient access over corporate interests, Australia maintains one of the most affordable drug markets in the world, making medications readily accessible and keeping out-of-pocket expenses low.

Japan has also adopted effective measures to control pharmaceutical costs. Its national health insurance system mandates price reviews for medications every two years, adjusting drug prices based on market data and cost-effectiveness. This regular adjustment ensures that the pricing remains fair and aligns with public healthcare goals, preventing drug costs from escalating unnecessarily. Japan's model balances innovation with public health, providing a system that meets the needs of patients while keeping healthcare expenditures in check.

These countries also emphasize transparency and accountability in drug pricing, with public reporting on how prices are set and adjusted over time. This transparency fosters public trust and enables stakeholders to hold pharmaceutical companies accountable for fair pricing. International organizations and coalitions also work to standardize pricing benchmarks across borders, encouraging ethical pricing and reducing the likelihood of price gouging.

This chapter provides an in-depth analysis of the price negotiation systems in Canada, Australia, and Japan, examining the impact of government healthcare systems on fair pricing, the role of transparency in promoting accountability, and international efforts to align drug costs with public welfare. By exploring how these global approaches might be adapted in the U.S., we can envision a healthcare system where affordability and access to medications are achievable goals, creating a more equitable and sustainable framework for American patients.

Price Negotiation Systems in Canada, Australia, and Japan

Price negotiation is a cornerstone of drug cost management in countries like Canada, Australia, and Japan, where government agencies are instrumental in setting prices that prioritize affordability and accessibility. In Canada, the Patented Medicine Prices Review Board (PMPRB) reviews the pricing of new drugs to ensure that they are not excessively high. The PMPRB evaluates each drug based on its therapeutic value and compares its price to those in other countries, establishing a fair price ceiling that protects Canadians from price gouging. By capping drug costs, the PMPRB helps maintain affordability, creating a system that mitigates the risk of inflated drug prices and ensures patients can access necessary medications without undue financial burden (Morgan et al., 2017).

Australia takes a similarly structured approach through its Pharmaceutical Benefits Scheme (PBS). This program negotiates drug prices directly with pharmaceutical companies, assessing both the cost-effectiveness and therapeutic value of each new medication. By basing prices on these factors, the PBS can subsidize medications, making them affordable for all Australians, regardless of income level. This system allows the government to carefully regulate which drugs are covered and to what extent, providing widespread access to essential medicines while keeping overall healthcare expenditures in check (Sweeny, 2014).

Japan's national health insurance system also relies heavily on regular price negotiations with pharmaceutical companies. Every two years, the

Japanese government reevaluates drug prices, adjusting them based on current market data and comparisons with international standards. This biennial price revision ensures that drug costs remain fair and reflect the actual value they provide to the healthcare system. By aligning drug prices with therapeutic benefit and cost-effectiveness, Japan's approach prevents unchecked price hikes and maintains consistency with global pricing, allowing patients access to medications at reasonable costs (Ikegami & Anderson, 2012).

This section examines how these negotiation frameworks effectively manage drug costs in Canada, Australia, and Japan. By setting fair prices through comprehensive reviews and regular adjustments, these countries illustrate how structured government intervention in drug pricing can create sustainable, affordable healthcare systems. Examples of these frameworks in action reveal their success in controlling prices, reducing out-of-pocket expenses, and maintaining equitable access to medications, offering valuable lessons for drug cost reform in other nations.

The Role of Government Healthcare Systems in Setting Fair Drug Prices

A key feature distinguishing international drug pricing strategies is the involvement of centralized healthcare systems, which leverage their purchasing power to negotiate fair and consistent prices for medications. In countries like Canada, Australia, and Japan, government healthcare systems serve as the primary purchasers of medications, giving them substantial negotiating power with pharmaceutical companies. This centralized structure contrasts sharply with the fragmented U.S. model, where multiple private insurers negotiate independently, resulting in inconsistent pricing and reduced bargaining power.

In Canada, the healthcare system works in conjunction with provincial drug plans to create a unified and coordinated pricing strategy. This collaboration ensures that drug prices are consistently regulated nationwide, preventing price disparities between regions and allowing Canadians broad access to medications at manageable costs. By acting as a collective buyer, Canada's healthcare system enhances affordability and protects citizens from the high out-of-pocket costs often seen in the U.S.

Australia's Pharmaceutical Benefits Scheme (PBS) operates under a similar single-payer framework, establishing baseline prices for essential medications. Through this model, the PBS not only ensures drug affordability for Australians but also carefully manages public health expenditures by evaluating each drug's cost-effectiveness and therapeutic value (Duckett & Willcox, 2015). The centralized approach enables Australia to contain drug costs while maintaining high standards of care and accessibility.

Japan's national health insurance system integrates its purchasing power with a structured process for routine price adjustments. Every two years, the Japanese government re-evaluates drug prices, adjusting them based on current economic conditions, international comparisons, and therapeutic value. This commitment to regular price revisions reflects Japan's focus on accessibility and financial sustainability, ensuring that citizens receive essential medications without incurring excessive expenses.

These centralized healthcare systems allow Canada, Australia, and Japan to provide essential medications at reasonable costs, minimizing financial burdens on individuals and maintaining a more equitable healthcare environment. In contrast, the U.S. system, with its multiple private insurers negotiating separately, lacks the unified purchasing power seen in other nations. This fragmentation results in inconsistent pricing and limited ability to leverage lower costs, underscoring the potential advantages of a more centralized model. By examining these international frameworks, we see how coordinated healthcare systems can achieve cost control, accessibility, and sustainability—offering valuable lessons for potential U.S. reforms.

International Efforts to Promote Transparency and Accountability in Pricing

Transparency and accountability in drug pricing are key priorities in many countries, fostering systems where pharmaceutical companies must justify their prices to regulatory bodies and the public. In the European Union, transparency directives mandate that pharmaceutical companies disclose their pricing methodologies and justify significant price increases. This open approach provides governments and the public with a clear view into the factors driving drug costs, allowing for scrutiny and reducing the risk of sudden, unwarranted price hikes (Vogler et al., 2017). By requiring transparency, EU nations create a regulatory environment that promotes accountability and deters opportunistic pricing.

Japan has also prioritized transparency, requiring pharmaceutical companies to submit comprehensive cost analyses when introducing new drugs. Additionally, Japan's healthcare system conducts regular reviews to ensure that drug prices reflect therapeutic value and remain competitive with international benchmarks. These biannual price evaluations not only adjust costs in line with economic and market conditions but also reinforce the government's commitment to fair and accessible healthcare. By aligning drug prices with therapeutic efficacy, Japan's system discourages arbitrary pricing and builds public trust in healthcare pricing policies.

Canada's approach has similarly evolved toward greater transparency, with the Patented Medicine Prices Review Board (PMPRB) actively monitoring and reporting on national price trends. The PMPRB analyzes pricing changes and evaluates significant price increases, providing the public with insights into cost dynamics and ensuring that price adjustments remain justified. This oversight helps to prevent unjustified costs and supports affordability across Canada's healthcare system.

These transparency initiatives contribute to more equitable healthcare systems by reducing the likelihood of price manipulation by pharmaceutical companies. By making pricing data available to both regulatory bodies and the public, these countries promote fair pricing practices and enable informed decision-making, fostering trust in the healthcare system. This section explores how transparency in drug pricing can deter unwarranted price hikes, encourage accountability, and create a more balanced healthcare environment where patients have access to essential medications without undue financial strain.

How Global Approaches Could Be Adapted for the U.S.

Although the U.S. healthcare system differs significantly from those in countries with single-payer or nationalized healthcare, there are lessons that could be adapted to create more affordable drug prices. Implementing a government-led price negotiation system, for example, could allow Medicare and other public health programs to leverage their purchasing power. Allowing Medicare to negotiate drug prices, similar to Canada's PMPRB or Australia's PBS, could significantly reduce costs for millions of Americans (Frank & Ginsburg, 2017).

Additionally, introducing transparency requirements for pharmaceutical companies could make pricing practices more accountable to the public. By mandating that drug manufacturers disclose pricing data and justify price increases, the U.S. could foster a system that prioritizes patient access and discourages profit-driven price hikes. Furthermore, a periodic review process, similar to Japan's biennial price adjustments, would enable the U.S. to ensure that drug prices remain fair and aligned with therapeutic value. This section explores these potential reforms and how they could be realistically implemented within the existing U.S. healthcare framework to provide better access and affordability for patients.

As drug prices continue to rise in the United States, the experiences of countries like Canada, Australia, and Japan offer valuable insights into creating a more equitable pharmaceutical landscape. By embracing price negotiation systems, leveraging the power of centralized healthcare, and promoting transparency, these countries have managed to provide affordable medications to their populations without sacrificing access to essential treatments. While the U.S. faces unique challenges, there are opportunities to adapt these global approaches, balancing innovation with affordability and ensuring that all Americans have access to life-saving medications. Addressing drug prices through these international lessons could pave the way for a more sustainable and patient-centered healthcare system.

Chapter 10

Attempts at Reform in the U.S.

As drug prices in the United States continue to soar, other countries have successfully implemented strategies to keep medications affordable and accessible for their citizens. Nations like Canada, Australia, and Japan have developed systems that leverage government negotiation, transparency, and centralized healthcare frameworks to balance cost and accessibility. These approaches contrast sharply with the U.S. model, where fragmented insurance structures and minimal government intervention often lead to high prices and inconsistent access. In this chapter, we explore these international models, examining how price negotiation, government healthcare systems, and accountability measures keep drug prices low. Through a detailed look at these global approaches, we uncover valuable insights that could guide U.S. policymakers in developing a more equitable and cost-effective healthcare system.

The Battle for Price Control: Policy Proposals and Failures

The high cost of prescription drugs in the United States has been a persistent issue, sparking repeated calls for reform aimed at making medications more accessible and affordable for American patients. Although there has been bipartisan support for initiatives to lower drug prices, many reform efforts have encountered significant political obstacles, often resulting in stalled progress or watered-down legislation. From proposals allowing Medicare to negotiate directly with pharmaceutical companies to provisions within the Affordable Care Act (ACA) designed to promote pricing transparency, numerous policy initiatives have sought to tackle the pharmaceutical pricing crisis. However, achieving meaningful change has proven challenging.

This chapter explores the history of U.S. policy efforts to control drug prices, beginning with the initial proposals to allow Medicare price negotiations—a concept widely supported by the public yet consistently blocked in Congress due to pharmaceutical industry opposition and lobbying. Although the ACA introduced measures intended to improve transparency, its impact on drug prices has been limited. Transparency alone has not translated into cost control, as pharmaceutical companies retain significant pricing power and leverage in a largely unregulated market.

Recent developments under the Biden administration have renewed focus on drug pricing reform. The administration has proposed allowing Medicare to negotiate the prices of certain high-cost medications directly, a major shift from previous policies. Additionally, new initiatives have aimed to cap out-of-pocket costs for seniors and reduce the impact of the Medicare "donut hole" coverage gap. On the state level, several states have passed legislation targeting drug price transparency, affordability, and even capping insulin costs, signaling a growing momentum for localized reform where federal initiatives have stalled.

This chapter also examines the political challenges that have historically hindered drug pricing reform, including the powerful influence of pharmaceutical lobbying, partisan divides, and the complexity of implementing changes within a decentralized, market-driven healthcare system. Despite these challenges, recent policy efforts provide valuable lessons. State-level actions, for instance, illustrate how targeted measures can mitigate high drug costs on a smaller scale, while broader federal proposals highlight the potential impact of structural reforms if they can overcome political resistance.

By analyzing past and current efforts, this chapter aims to outline key lessons for future policy approaches, emphasizing the need for persistent advocacy, bipartisan support, and innovative solutions that prioritize patient access and affordability. As drug prices continue to strain consumers and healthcare systems alike, these lessons serve as critical touchpoints for building a healthcare framework where essential medications are within reach for all Americans.

Overview of U.S. Policy Efforts to Lower Drug Prices

Over the past two decades, numerous policy initiatives have aimed to address the high cost of prescription drugs, though with mixed results. Among the most prominent proposals has been to grant Medicare the authority to negotiate prices directly with pharmaceutical companies. Currently, Medicare—a major driver of U.S. healthcare spending—is legally barred from price negotiations, a restriction that critics argue severely limits the government's bargaining power and contributes to escalating costs (Huang & Catlin, 2021). While various legislative efforts have sought to lift this restriction, none have yet succeeded.

The Affordable Care Act (ACA) of 2010 implemented measures intended to reduce drug costs, including expanding access to generic drugs and closing the "donut hole" gap in Medicare Part D coverage. Although these provisions provided some cost relief for consumers, they did not tackle the core pricing control wielded by pharmaceutical companies, leaving fundamental pricing issues largely intact (Oberlander, 2010).

Other legislative efforts, such as the CREATES Act, targeted anti-competitive practices designed to delay the market entry of generics, with the goal of increasing affordability through competition. However, while the CREATES Act addressed some barriers, its overall impact has been limited, and significant pricing challenges persist.

This section examines these key policy efforts, analyzing their intended goals, specific measures, and the degree to which they have alleviated the financial burden of high drug prices for patients. Each initiative sheds light on both the potential and limitations of legislative approaches to reducing drug costs, underscoring the need for further reform in the U.S. pharmaceutical market.

The Political Roadblocks: Why Reforms Have Failed or Stalled

Despite widespread support for reducing drug prices, political obstacles have consistently hindered progress. Pharmaceutical companies wield significant lobbying power, spending hundreds of millions of dollars annually to influence policy and protect their pricing structures (Sachs, 2021). Organizations like the Pharmaceutical Research and Manufacturers of America (PhRMA) have been instrumental in blocking legislation that could harm the industry's profits. This lobbying power, combined with substantial campaign contributions to both parties, has resulted in a gridlocked policy environment where few reforms gain enough traction to pass.

Additionally, ideological differences over the role of government in regulating the private sector complicate reform efforts. While some legislators advocate for government intervention to control prices, others argue that price regulation stifles innovation and interferes with the free market. These conflicting perspectives contribute to legislative inertia, as reform proposals are often compromised or abandoned to satisfy opposing factions within Congress (Mazzucato, 2018). This section examines the powerful influence of the pharmaceutical lobby and the ideological divides that have prevented meaningful drug pricing reform in the United States.

Recent Developments: Biden Administration and State-Level Initiatives

The Biden administration has actively sought to address rising drug prices, introducing several initiatives aimed at making medications more affordable for Americans. In 2021, the administration announced a significant proposal allowing Medicare to negotiate prices for specific high-cost medications—a policy that, if implemented, would mark a major shift in how the government addresses prescription drug costs. By enabling Medicare, which represents a substantial share of U.S. healthcare spending, to negotiate directly with pharmaceutical companies, this policy could drive down prices for some of the most expensive medications and put pressure on the broader pharmaceutical market to adjust pricing practices (Biden, 2021).

Alongside Medicare negotiation rights, the Biden administration's plan includes capping out-of-pocket expenses for Medicare beneficiaries, directly reducing financial burdens for millions of elderly and disabled Americans who often struggle with the high costs of their medications. Additionally, the proposal seeks to implement penalties on pharmaceutical companies that increase prices faster than the rate of inflation. This inflation cap could prevent drug prices from escalating rapidly year over year, helping to maintain more predictable costs for consumers. While these measures have gained traction and raised hopes for real change, they still face strong resistance from industry groups. Pharmaceutical companies and lobbying organizations, which argue that such regulations could stifle innovation and reduce the funds available for drug research, are working to weaken or block these policies, making the path through Congress a challenging one.

At the state level, several states have stepped up with their own reforms to tackle high drug prices, addressing the issue where federal initiatives have been delayed or limited. For example, California introduced the CalRx program, which aims to produce affordable generic medications as alternatives to more expensive brand-name drugs (California Department of Public Health, 2020). By manufacturing its own line of generic drugs, California is pioneering a unique approach to circumvent the high costs often associated with brand-name pharmaceuticals, providing residents with access to essential medications at a reduced price.

Other states, such as Maryland and New York, have passed legislation focused on increasing transparency in drug pricing and restricting excessive price hikes on essential drugs. These measures mandate that drug companies disclose pricing information and justify price increases, allowing for greater public and regulatory oversight. While these state initiatives may not directly lower drug prices across the board, they create pressure for pharmaceutical companies to be more accountable in their pricing strategies and offer a potential model for broader national reforms.

Together, these federal and state-level efforts illustrate a growing determination to address the high costs of prescription drugs, albeit within the constraints of political and industry opposition. This section explores these recent policy developments, evaluating their potential impact on drug pricing and the challenges they face in implementation. While federal initiatives have the potential for sweeping changes, state-level policies serve as innovative experiments that, if successful, could inspire and inform broader national reforms. However, significant hurdles remain, from powerful pharmaceutical lobbying to ideological divides in Congress, all of which complicate the path toward meaningful, widespread reform.

Lessons Learned from Past and Ongoing Reform Efforts

The repeated failure of drug pricing reform in the United States offers several important lessons for future policy efforts. First, the power of lobbying underscores the need for transparency and limits on campaign contributions from pharmaceutical companies, as financial influence plays a substantial role in policy outcomes. Efforts to reform drug prices may be more successful with stronger ethics regulations around lobbying and campaign finance.

Second, incremental reforms, such as those at the state level, may provide a viable path forward. While federal reform has proven challenging, state-level initiatives can serve as testing grounds for policies that, if successful, could be adopted nationwide. Finally, bipartisan support is essential for durable policy solutions. By framing drug pricing reform as a matter of public health rather than partisanship, future efforts may stand a better chance of overcoming legislative gridlock (Kesselheim & Avorn, 2021). This section reflects on the successes and failures of past reforms, offering insights for building more effective policies in the future.

The fight to control drug prices in the United States is a challenging, ongoing battle shaped by powerful lobbying interests, ideological divides, and policy setbacks. Despite the promise of reforms from Medicare negotiations to state-led initiatives, meaningful progress has been limited, leaving millions of Americans to bear the burden of high drug costs. Examining recent efforts by the Biden administration and innovative state programs highlights potential paths forward, though the hurdles remain significant. By learning from past reform attempts and addressing political barriers, policymakers may finally develop strategies that bring relief to patients while preserving the innovation and competitiveness of the pharmaceutical industry.

Chapter 11

Possible Solutions for America

The issue of high drug prices in the United States has reached a tipping point, with millions of Americans facing financial strain—or even risking their health—due to the cost of essential medications. Although previous efforts to reform drug pricing have struggled against political and economic barriers, the urgency of the crisis demands new, bold approaches. This chapter explores practical solutions that could finally bring relief, from empowering Medicare to negotiate drug prices to promoting competition through generics and biosimilars. We also examine strategies to reduce the influence of Big Pharma's lobbying and leverage public support for reform. By considering these comprehensive measures, we can identify a path forward that balances affordability with innovation, putting the needs of American patients first.

Charting a Path Forward: How America Can Fix Its Drug Pricing Problem

The escalating cost of prescription drugs in the United States has ignited a widespread debate on reforming the pharmaceutical landscape to ensure greater affordability and access for patients. Although previous efforts to control drug prices have often faced political resistance and structural challenges, there is now a growing consensus that targeted policies could reduce costs without stifling innovation. This chapter explores a range of practical policy recommendations aimed at addressing high drug prices, providing a roadmap for creating a more affordable and accessible drug market in the U.S.

One of the most widely supported proposals involves allowing Medicare to negotiate directly with pharmaceutical companies on drug prices, a practice already implemented by many other high-income nations. Granting Medicare this authority could significantly reduce prices for high-cost medications, given Medicare's substantial purchasing power. Additionally, instituting price controls or caps on certain essential medications, such as insulin, would provide immediate financial relief for patients who rely on these drugs. This approach has already shown promise in states where insulin price caps have been enacted, suggesting a scalable model for federal action.

Expanding the use of generic drugs and biosimilars is another effective strategy for reducing drug costs. By streamlining the approval process for generics and biosimilars and encouraging their adoption, policymakers could increase competition in the market, driving down prices for patients. This would involve regulatory reforms that simplify pathways for generics and biosimilars to reach consumers more quickly, as well as incentives for healthcare providers and insurers to prioritize these cost-effective alternatives.

Another critical area for reform is the influence of pharmaceutical lobbying on drug pricing policy. Pharmaceutical companies spend millions each year on lobbying efforts, which can impede meaningful legislative progress. Implementing measures to limit lobbying and increase transparency in campaign contributions could help reduce this influence and allow for more patient-centered policy development. Additionally, increased public pressure and consumer advocacy have proven powerful in shaping policy, as seen in recent efforts to cap out-of-pocket costs and enhance drug price transparency. By galvanizing public support, advocates can bring accountability to lawmakers and create momentum for reform.

By examining these policy recommendations—Medicare price negotiations, price controls, expanded use of generics and biosimilars, limitations on lobbying, and the mobilization of public pressure—this chapter charts a path forward for reshaping the U.S. pharmaceutical market. With a combination of regulatory reform, market-driven solutions, and public advocacy, the United States has the potential to create a healthcare landscape where drug prices are both manageable and equitable, prioritizing patient welfare alongside pharmaceutical innovation.

Policy Recommendations to Curb High Drug Prices

To effectively address high drug prices, policymakers need a multifaceted strategy that combines regulation, increased market competition, and robust consumer protections. A central policy recommendation is to empower the government to negotiate drug prices, particularly within the Medicare program. Granting Medicare this negotiation power would allow the government to use its considerable purchasing leverage to secure lower prices, as observed in other developed countries with similar programs (Anderson et al., 2021). Such negotiations could yield substantial cost savings for patients and taxpayers alike, especially for high-cost medications frequently used by seniors and individuals with chronic conditions.

Another approach involves implementing price caps or limits on annual price increases for essential drugs. By establishing caps, policymakers can prevent pharmaceutical companies from making arbitrary or excessive price hikes on medications that patients depend on, ensuring greater price stability and predictability.

Incentivizing the development and market entry of generic drugs is also a critical component of this strategy. Expanding incentives and streamlining approval pathways for generics and biosimilars would enhance market competition, helping to drive down drug prices as affordable alternatives become more readily available. This approach can be complemented by shortening patent exclusivity periods, which would reduce the time that brand-name drugs maintain monopoly pricing, allowing generics to enter the market sooner and contribute to cost reductions (Kesselheim et al., 2019).

Promoting price transparency across the pharmaceutical supply chain is another essential reform. Transparency laws would require pharmaceutical companies to disclose the primary factors driving their pricing decisions, offering the public and policymakers insight into the true cost of drug production and distribution. This transparency would encourage accountability, as companies would need to justify price increases, making it more challenging to engage in opaque pricing practices.

This section outlines these critical policy options, examining the potential impact of Medicare price negotiations, price caps, increased generic competition, reduced patent exclusivity, and price transparency on drug affordability in the U.S. By evaluating these approaches, we can better understand how each could contribute to a more equitable pharmaceutical market, creating a healthcare environment where drug costs are manageable and access to medications is prioritized.

The Potential of Medicare Price Negotiations and Price Controls

Allowing Medicare to negotiate drug prices holds transformative potential for the U.S. pharmaceutical landscape. However, under current law, Medicare is prohibited from directly negotiating prices with pharmaceutical companies, leaving it highly vulnerable to drug manufacturers' pricing strategies. As a result, Medicare, one of the largest purchasers of medications in the U.S., lacks the leverage to secure cost reductions for its beneficiaries, often paying significantly more than other high-income nations for the same medications. Implementing a policy that enables Medicare negotiation could lead to substantial savings for millions of Americans, drawing from successful models in countries like Germany and the United Kingdom, where national health services negotiate directly with pharmaceutical companies to secure lower prices (Kanavos et al., 2011). With such a policy, Medicare could potentially save billions of dollars annually, easing financial pressure on both the program and its beneficiaries.

However, despite broad public support, numerous attempts to empower Medicare with negotiating authority have failed due to substantial political resistance, particularly from pharmaceutical lobbying groups and some policymakers concerned about potential impacts on industry innovation. The pharmaceutical industry argues that price negotiations would reduce revenue and stymie the development of new drugs. Yet, other high-income countries demonstrate that robust negotiation practices can coexist with active pharmaceutical innovation. The resistance to this reform highlights a disconnect between public interest in affordability and industry influence over policy decisions.

Beyond Medicare negotiation, introducing price controls on select high-cost drugs could further address the issue of exorbitant pricing. Many countries, such as Canada, use regulatory bodies to assess the therapeutic value and set fair pricing for new drugs, ensuring that prices align with the benefits they offer (Morgan et al., 2017). By contrast, the U.S. pharmaceutical market operates with limited price regulation, allowing companies to set high prices without government oversight. Although price controls face significant opposition in the U.S.—with critics arguing they would disrupt free-market dynamics—proponents believe they are necessary to prevent unregulated pricing power from compromising access to essential medications.

The potential benefits of Medicare negotiations and targeted price controls are clear: these mechanisms could provide price stability, reduce out-of-pocket expenses, and help contain overall healthcare costs. However, the limitations are also significant. Political opposition, heavy lobbying from pharmaceutical companies, and concerns about impacts on innovation create formidable roadblocks to implementing these strategies. The strength of the pharmaceutical industry's lobbying power has consistently blocked policy efforts aimed at addressing high drug prices, with the industry spending hundreds of millions annually to influence legislation. Additionally, without comprehensive reform, Medicare negotiation and price controls alone may not address other underlying factors, such as high deductibles and insurance-related barriers, that also limit patient access.

This section explores the mechanisms, potential outcomes, and challenges of Medicare negotiations and price controls, weighing the significant benefits against the practical and political limitations. By examining these issues, we can better understand why such strategies, while promising in theory, face major hurdles in the U.S. and why a multifaceted approach—including regulatory, market, and public pressure initiatives—may be necessary to bring about meaningful change in the American pharmaceutical market.

Expanding the Role of Generic Drugs and Biosimilars in the U.S.

Generic drugs and biosimilars play a critical role in reducing drug prices by introducing competition into the pharmaceutical market. In theory, the availability of generics and biosimilars should drive down prices as more affordable alternatives to brand-name drugs become accessible. However, in the U.S., the market entry of these alternatives is often significantly delayed due to patent extensions, exclusivity periods, and lengthy legal challenges initiated by brand-name manufacturers. These barriers allow brand-name companies to extend their market dominance and pricing power well beyond the initial patent expiration, keeping costs high for patients and limiting options for affordable care (Grabowski et al., 2016).

Policymakers could address these delays by revisiting and revising patent laws to restrict practices that extend patent life, such as "evergreening," which involves making minor modifications to a drug solely to renew its exclusivity period. Reducing these exclusivity periods would encourage competition sooner, allowing generics and biosimilars to enter the market faster and provide more affordable options for patients. Additionally, expediting the approval process for generics at the FDA could minimize the time required to bring these drugs to consumers.

Biosimilars, which are biologically similar versions of complex biologic drugs, hold particular promise in reducing costs for high-priced treatments, especially in fields like oncology, immunology, and rare diseases. Unlike small-molecule generics, which are chemically identical to their brand-name counterparts, biosimilars are derived from living cells and are thus not identical to the original biologic but are highly similar in terms of efficacy and safety. Due to their complexity, biosimilars often face additional regulatory and manufacturing hurdles, which contribute to higher development costs and slower market entry.

Countries like Germany and other European nations have embraced biosimilars, achieving substantial savings in healthcare without compromising patient care. For instance, Germany's strong biosimilar adoption has been supported by government policies that incentivize healthcare providers to prescribe biosimilars, resulting in millions saved annually. Studies have shown that the adoption of biosimilars has led to a 20-30% reduction in prices for biologic treatments, which provides a clear example of the potential financial benefits (Tabernero et al., 2017).

Streamlining the FDA's approval process for biosimilars and strengthening incentives for their production could replicate these savings in the U.S. Policymakers could incentivize the manufacturing of biosimilars by providing tax credits, grants, or market entry assistance for companies willing to invest in biosimilar production. Such incentives would encourage greater competition and help biosimilars gain a stronger foothold in the U.S. market. Additionally, introducing guidelines that encourage healthcare providers to consider biosimilars as a first-line treatment option when appropriate could further bolster their adoption, making it easier for patients to access affordable, life-saving therapies.

This section explored key strategies for increasing the availability and adoption of generics and biosimilars, drawing on successful international examples. These strategies underscore the potential of generics and biosimilars to lower drug prices across the healthcare system, reduce out-of-pocket costs for patients, and ease the financial burden on insurance providers and public health programs.

How to Break the Lobbying Stranglehold of Big Pharma

The formidable influence of pharmaceutical lobbying presents a significant barrier to drug pricing reform in the United States. Each year, the pharmaceutical industry spends hundreds of millions of dollars on lobbying to block, dilute, or delay proposed reforms, often hiring former government officials who leverage their insider knowledge and networks to advocate for industry interests (Ornstein & Weber, 2018). This revolving door between government and industry reinforces Big Pharma's hold over drug pricing policy, frequently prioritizing corporate profits over patient access and affordability.

Addressing this issue will require substantial legislative action to reduce the industry's sway over policymakers. One approach is to introduce stricter regulations on lobbying practices, mandating transparency in lobbying expenditures and disclosing all financial relationships between pharmaceutical companies and legislators. Additionally, restrictions on the revolving door could help curb conflicts of interest by limiting the ability of former government officials to move directly into influential industry roles, where they often lobby on behalf of the very companies they once regulated.

Campaign finance reform is another critical element in reducing Big Pharma's influence over drug policy. Currently, pharmaceutical companies and their political action committees (PACs) contribute significant amounts to political campaigns, ensuring favorable relationships with key legislators on both sides of the aisle. By imposing limits on campaign contributions from pharmaceutical companies and their PACs, lawmakers could help diminish this outsized influence, fostering a legislative environment that prioritizes public welfare over corporate agendas (Sachs, 2021).

Implementing these reforms would require bipartisan support and a commitment to creating a balanced healthcare system that serves patient interests rather than corporate profits. Although such changes may face initial resistance, the long-term benefits of reducing lobbying influence could reshape U.S. drug policy, creating a more patient-centered approach to drug pricing and access.

This section explores the pharmaceutical industry's current lobbying practices, including the scope of financial influence and the impact of the revolving door on policy outcomes. By outlining potential reforms—such as transparency mandates, revolving door restrictions, and campaign finance limitations—this discussion highlights pathways for lawmakers to break Big Pharma's stronghold over drug policy, setting the stage for more balanced and accessible healthcare reforms.

The Role of Public Pressure and Grassroots Movements

Public pressure has proven effective in driving policy changes across various sectors, and the pharmaceutical industry is no exception. Grassroots movements, such as Patients for Affordable Drugs and Lower Drug Prices Now, have successfully raised awareness of the impact of high drug prices and lobbied for legislative action. Public campaigns highlighting the human costs of high prices have not only generated media attention but also influenced policymakers to consider reforms previously deemed politically risky (Sachs, 2021).

Increasing public awareness of the pharmaceutical industry's pricing practices and lobbying efforts can galvanize citizens to demand change. Tools like social media and public demonstrations amplify these voices, encouraging policymakers to take action. This section discusses the role of public pressure in reshaping the drug pricing landscape, examining how grassroots movements have influenced recent legislative initiatives and advocating for increased public involvement in the fight for affordable medications.

Addressing the U.S. drug pricing problem will require comprehensive reforms that involve policy changes, increased competition, and a reduction in industry influence over legislation. By embracing Medicare price negotiations, supporting the entry of generics and biosimilars, and implementing lobbying and campaign finance reforms, the U.S. can begin to create a more equitable pharmaceutical market. Furthermore, public pressure and grassroots movements will play a crucial role in sustaining momentum for these changes, holding policymakers accountable to prioritize patient welfare over corporate profits. These solutions collectively offer a path forward for reducing drug costs and ensuring that all Americans have access to affordable, life-saving medications.

Chapter 12

Why Neither Democrats nor Republicans Will Ever Fix Drug Prices

The escalating cost of prescription drugs has long been a point of frustration for Americans, yet meaningful reform remains elusive. Despite rhetoric from both Democrats and Republicans promising to lower drug prices, neither party has managed to enact lasting change. At the heart of this inaction lies the powerful influence of Big Pharma—a well-funded, politically savvy industry that spends millions on campaign contributions and lobbying each year. This chapter examines the symbiotic relationship between the pharmaceutical industry and both major political parties, illustrating why substantial drug pricing reform is unlikely as long as Big Pharma's financial interests align with campaign finance dynamics. Additionally, it highlights how the American taxpayer often remains unaware of this dynamic, manipulated by political narratives that fail to address the root issues in drug pricing.

The Power of Big Pharma's Campaign Contributions

Big Pharma's influence in Washington is powered by its vast financial resources, strategically directed into lobbying and campaign contributions to secure favorable policies. Each election cycle, pharmaceutical companies and their political action committees (PACs) make substantial contributions to candidates across both the

Democratic and Republican parties. This strategy is intentionally bipartisan: by supporting candidates from both parties, Big Pharma ensures its interests are safeguarded, regardless of which side gains power. The scale of these contributions is staggering. The pharmaceutical industry routinely spends more on lobbying than nearly any other sector, with annual expenditures often exceeding $300 million. This extensive financial backing solidifies the industry's standing in the halls of power, enabling it to shape legislation, maintain favorable policies, and uphold high drug pricing strategies (OpenSecrets, 2022; Ornstein & Weber, 2018).

A key element of Big Pharma's strategy involves targeting contributions based on specific policy stances. Pharmaceutical companies carefully track the legislative positions of lawmakers, prioritizing support for those who are sympathetic to industry interests or are willing to oppose significant pricing reforms. This flexibility allows Big Pharma to pivot its contributions based on the political climate, ensuring that no matter which party proposes drug pricing reforms, the industry can quickly redirect funds to support the opposition or primary challengers who align with its goals (Sachs, 2021). This practice acts as a powerful deterrent against aggressive drug pricing reform, as lawmakers know that advocating for stringent regulations or price controls could result in losing essential campaign funding and encountering well-financed opposition.

This pervasive influence generates a bipartisan hesitancy to pursue meaningful changes that could disrupt the pharmaceutical industry's profit margins, despite the potential benefit for millions of Americans. Even when drug pricing reforms have broad public support, such as allowing Medicare to negotiate drug prices, the significant lobbying power of Big Pharma often prevails, leading to watered-down proposals or outright blockages in Congress. Lawmakers, aware of the substantial financial stakes, are reluctant to alienate a major contributor that can swiftly fund their opponents or influence upcoming elections. The result is a political environment where the cost of drugs remains high, and comprehensive reform is consistently delayed, as the pharmaceutical industry prioritizes its profitability over the welfare of the public.

This financial dominance allows Big Pharma to maintain a firm hold on U.S. healthcare policy, influencing both parties to avoid drastic changes that could cut into industry profits. The fear of facing a well-funded adversary, paired with the allure of continued campaign contributions, keeps lawmakers from pushing for the reforms that many American patients desperately need. In this way, Big Pharma not only protects its interests but also shapes a legislative status quo that ensures its pricing strategies remain intact. The consequences of this influence are felt by millions of Americans who struggle to afford essential medications while lawmakers fail to deliver the reforms they are promised.

The "Revolving Door" and Political Influence

Beyond campaign contributions, Big Pharma has perfected the "revolving door" strategy, a practice where former government officials are hired into high-paying industry positions and, conversely, industry executives transition into influential roles within government agencies. This flow of personnel back and forth between the pharmaceutical industry and government solidifies Big Pharma's connections within the political and regulatory spheres, enabling the industry to exert a more profound influence on drug policy (Ornstein & Weber, 2018). Former government officials, once employed by the pharmaceutical sector, bring with them invaluable insider knowledge and networks, using these resources to lobby more effectively for policies that benefit the industry.

The revolving door creates a mutually beneficial relationship that ultimately disadvantages American patients. Former regulatory officials often become industry lobbyists, advisers, or executives, leveraging the access they gained while in public office. Meanwhile, when pharmaceutical executives take on government roles, they bring with them a strong bias toward industry interests, influencing policy in ways that protect pharmaceutical profits. This flow of personnel back and forth reinforces Big Pharma's influence on both political parties, as former officials maintain connections with current lawmakers and bureaucrats, subtly swaying policy decisions toward industry priorities.

The impact of the revolving door is not only about the exchange of personnel but also about the consistent alignment of policies with pharmaceutical industry goals. For example, when former Food and Drug Administration (FDA) or Department of Health and Human Services (HHS) officials join pharmaceutical companies, they are often tasked with navigating or lobbying against regulations that would otherwise control drug prices or expedite the approval of generics. Their previous government experience gives them a unique advantage, enabling them to exploit policy loopholes, understand regulatory weaknesses, and design strategies that can effectively delay market competition. This cycle ensures that even well-intentioned drug pricing reform efforts encounter obstacles from within the government itself, as former regulators use their insider expertise to advocate for corporate interests, further stymying any progress toward affordable medication (OpenSecrets, 2022).

The revolving door's influence is pervasive and long-lasting, fostering a policy environment where pharmaceutical interests are prioritized over patient affordability. High-ranking officials who have previously worked within the FDA or other healthcare agencies often maintain close connections with their former colleagues, creating a feedback loop that reinforces industry-friendly policies. In many cases, these former officials have direct access to lawmakers, allowing them to quietly shape drug policy in ways that align with the industry's financial goals. This deeply entrenched cycle of influence effectively blocks reform from the inside, allowing Big Pharma to maintain high drug prices and avoid significant policy changes that could threaten its profits.

For the American public, the revolving door represents a significant barrier to achieving meaningful healthcare reform. The practice fosters a closed-loop system where the industry's priorities are protected by a network of former government officials, current regulators, and political allies. As long as the revolving door remains open, Big Pharma's influence will continue to dominate, leaving even the most well-meaning policy efforts hindered by industry-driven interests embedded within the government.

Rhetoric vs. Reality: Why Campaign Promises Fall Short

Both parties frequently acknowledge the financial burden of high drug prices on American families, with candidates from both sides often making campaign promises to address the issue. Once elected, however, these promises rarely translate into substantial policy changes. Democrats, for example, might propose allowing Medicare to negotiate drug prices, while Republicans often advocate for market competition as a solution. Yet, these proposals seldom lead to concrete reforms that would meaningfully lower drug prices. A significant reason for this lack of progress is both parties' financial dependence on Big Pharma contributions, which creates a strong disincentive to enact policies that would genuinely impact pharmaceutical profits (Sachs, 2021).

One of the most widely supported reforms is Medicare negotiation, a policy that holds the potential to significantly lower prescription drug prices by leveraging Medicare's purchasing power. Despite this support, both parties have repeatedly failed to pass legislation enabling such negotiations. Attempts to regulate drug prices or cap out-of-pocket costs face a similar fate, often stalling in Congress or being significantly watered down to the point that their impact is minimal. Behind closed doors, pharmaceutical lobbyists play a critical role in shaping the outcome of these legislative efforts. Through targeted lobbying, they work to undermine reform proposals, often by influencing specific aspects of the legislation. In many cases, these lobbyists secure subtle changes or include clauses that effectively neutralize the intended impact, ensuring that pharmaceutical profits remain protected (Kanavos et al., 2011).

This dynamic creates a legislative environment where the appearance of progress is prioritized over meaningful action. Lawmakers, aware of the public's demand for lower drug prices, may propose reforms that sound impactful, yet behind the scenes, lobbyists influence the language of these bills to maintain loopholes or reduce the measures' effectiveness. For example, attempts to cap insulin costs or increase price transparency may initially seem promising, but amendments or vague language added to the bills can significantly weaken their enforcement. In this way, both parties can claim they are addressing high drug prices while allowing Big Pharma to continue its pricing practices largely unchecked.

The underlying financial dependency on Big Pharma contributions ensures that both parties remain cautious about pushing reforms that could truly threaten pharmaceutical profits. Lawmakers are aware that aggressive reform could lead to a withdrawal of campaign funds, or worse, an influx of Big Pharma dollars into their opponents' campaigns. This risk discourages them from pursuing meaningful changes that would challenge the pharmaceutical industry's influence, resulting in a continuous cycle of high drug prices and failed promises.

Ultimately, the result is a political stalemate where both parties publicly champion drug pricing reform but lack the political will to enact substantive change. This reliance on Big Pharma's financial backing undermines the public's trust in the legislative process and leaves millions of Americans burdened by unaffordable prescription drug costs.

The High Cost of Opposition: How Big Pharma Protects Its Interests

Pharmaceutical companies have made it abundantly clear that any legislative efforts challenging their pricing structures will be met with swift and aggressive opposition. If a political party or individual lawmaker proposes policies that could threaten Big Pharma's profit margins, the industry has the resources to pivot its financial support to opponents or well-funded primary challengers, placing immense pressure on legislators to avoid pursuing meaningful reforms. This capability to redirect financial resources acts as a powerful deterrent, discouraging lawmakers from backing any proposals that might truly curb industry profits (Sachs, 2021).

The pharmaceutical industry has a variety of tactics to dissuade lawmakers from pushing reform. For example, when legislators introduce measures that limit patent extensions or enhance transparency in drug pricing, Big Pharma can retaliate by funding negative ad campaigns against those individuals, effectively tarnishing their public image. These campaigns can portray reform-minded lawmakers as anti-business or frame their initiatives as harmful to the economy and public health. Additionally, pharmaceutical companies can directly fund primary challengers who oppose these reforms, pressuring incumbents to abandon potentially impactful legislation in favor of political security. In many cases, the mere threat of losing industry support or facing an influx of negative ads is enough to dissuade legislators from pursuing reform, particularly when they know that Big Pharma has the financial power to significantly influence their re-election outcomes (Morgan et al., 2017).

This high cost of opposition ensures that any serious attempt to regulate drug prices comes with substantial political risks. Lawmakers who persist in advocating for change may find themselves isolated, as Big Pharma uses its financial influence to protect the status quo. This tactic has helped the industry maintain its pricing power, allowing it to continue charging Americans some of the highest drug prices in the world. By targeting reform-minded lawmakers and aligning itself with political figures who support its agenda, Big Pharma not only preserves its influence but also creates a political environment where substantive reform becomes nearly impossible.

Ultimately, the pharmaceutical industry's willingness to weaponize its resources in defense of its interests contributes to a political climate where meaningful drug pricing reform is perpetually out of reach. The consequences are felt acutely by American patients, who continue to struggle with rising prescription costs while lawmakers, facing financial and political pressure from Big Pharma, remain hesitant to push for the changes that could alleviate this burden.

The Public as Political Pawns: The Role of Voter Misinformation

Amid this complex landscape of political and financial maneuvering, the American public often remains largely unaware of the depth of Big Pharma's influence over drug policy. Both Democrats and Republicans are well aware that high drug prices are a significant issue for voters, and they frequently leverage this concern as a campaign talking point, promising to tackle rising costs and make medications more affordable. Yet, once in office, these promises often dissolve, as party leaders prioritize the pharmaceutical industry's financial backing over meaningful reform. This dynamic leaves American taxpayers as pawns in a political system where neither party is genuinely motivated to take on Big Pharma.

Without sufficient transparency or public education on the pharmaceutical industry's influence, the public often accepts campaign rhetoric at face value, trusting in politicians' intentions to lower drug prices without realizing the systemic obstacles that prevent these promises from materializing. The lack of public awareness about Big Pharma's role in shaping drug policy and blocking reform allows the industry to maintain its influence with minimal resistance. As a result, Americans continue to pay some of the highest drug prices in the world, while the true reasons for unaffordable medications remain hidden behind a veil of lobbying, campaign contributions, and political influence.

This lack of transparency perpetuates a cycle in which voters, despite holding strong opinions about the need for affordable healthcare, are left in the dark about the reasons their concerns go unaddressed. Without broader awareness and accountability, Big Pharma maintains its firm grip on policy, ensuring that the structural causes of high drug prices remain largely unchallenged, leaving Americans paying the price.

The Result: A Stalemate in Drug Pricing Reform

The high cost of prescription drugs in the United States is a complex issue influenced by various factors, including the significant political power wielded by the pharmaceutical industry. Both major political parties, Democrats and Republicans, have expressed concerns over drug prices and have proposed reforms. However, substantial changes have been elusive, leading to speculation about the underlying reasons for this inertia.

The pharmaceutical industry is among the top spenders on lobbying activities in Washington, D.C. In 2020, the industry spent over $309 million on lobbying efforts, with the Pharmaceutical Research and Manufacturers of America (PhRMA) contributing significantly to this expenditure.

These funds are strategically distributed to both political parties, ensuring that the industry's interests are well-represented, regardless of the prevailing political climate.

Campaign contributions are another avenue through which Big Pharma exerts influence. By financially supporting candidates from both parties, pharmaceutical companies aim to secure favorable policies and protect their profit margins. This bipartisan funding approach ensures that, irrespective of which party is in power, the industry's interests remain safeguarded.

The "revolving door" between government agencies and the pharmaceutical industry further solidifies Big Pharma's influence over drug policy. Former government officials often transition into roles within the pharmaceutical sector, leveraging their insider knowledge and connections to advance industry objectives. This practice can lead to regulatory decisions that favor pharmaceutical companies, sometimes at the expense of public health interests.

The financial dependencies and intertwined relationships between Big Pharma and political entities create substantial obstacles to meaningful drug pricing reform. Efforts to allow Medicare to negotiate drug prices, implement price controls, or increase market competition often face resistance not only from the industry but also from legislators who may be influenced by pharmaceutical contributions. This dynamic contributes to the United States having some of the highest prescription drug prices globally, with minimal prospects for significant reductions in the near future.

The entrenched influence of the pharmaceutical industry in American politics, through extensive lobbying, campaign contributions, and the revolving door, has created a landscape where both major parties are hesitant to enact substantial reforms that could jeopardize industry profits. Consequently, American consumers continue to bear the burden of high prescription drug costs, with limited hope for transformative change under the current system.

The Path Forward: Breaking Big Pharma's Hold on Policy

Meaningful drug pricing reform will necessitate fundamental changes in campaign financing and the relationship between the pharmaceutical industry and lawmakers. Reforming campaign finance laws to reduce or outright ban corporate contributions from pharmaceutical companies is essential to curbing Big Pharma's influence over drug policy. Stricter restrictions on the "revolving door"—the practice of government officials transitioning into industry positions and vice versa—could further limit the industry's power, as it would prevent former regulators and lawmakers from lobbying on behalf of pharmaceutical interests immediately after leaving office. These steps are critical to weakening the hold pharmaceutical interests currently have on the legislative process; without them, both major political parties will likely remain ensnared in a cycle where policy decisions favor corporate interests over the public's health needs.

Public advocacy and transparency are crucial in the interim. Increased public pressure through grassroots campaigns, coupled with a media spotlight on the influence of Big Pharma, can expose the role the industry plays in obstructing reform. This heightened awareness can shift the narrative and help create accountability, pushing policymakers to prioritize patient welfare above corporate profits. Media scrutiny and advocacy groups can encourage lawmakers to resist pharmaceutical funding and support genuine reforms that place patients' needs at the forefront.

Ultimately, until the political system reduces its dependency on Big Pharma's financial backing, neither Democrats nor Republicans are likely to implement the comprehensive drug pricing reforms that American patients urgently need. Pharmaceutical companies have significant influence over both parties through extensive lobbying efforts and substantial campaign contributions, creating a political landscape in which industry interests often take precedence over consumer welfare. This financial backing gives Big Pharma a seat at the policymaking table, allowing it to shape legislation, stifle reforms, and protect profit margins, even as public outcry over high drug prices grows.

For genuine reform to take place, it would require both parties to adopt stricter regulations on lobbying practices and campaign financing, diminishing the hold that pharmaceutical companies have over elected officials. Without this structural change, attempts at reform are often diluted or stalled in Congress, as lawmakers face pressure from industry lobbyists to prioritize corporate interests over those of consumers. Until these ties are loosened, political leaders are unlikely to challenge the status quo in a way that could meaningfully lower drug prices, leaving patients to bear the financial burden of high medication costs.

The need for systemic change extends beyond individual reforms to a fundamental reevaluation of how political influence is financed and regulated. Only by addressing the entrenched dependency on Big Pharma's financial support can legislators hope to create a healthcare system that genuinely prioritizes patient access, affordability, and long-term public health.

Chapter 13

Big Pharma and Insurance Companies

The intricate relationship between Big Pharma and insurance companies plays a pivotal role in shaping drug prices and overall healthcare costs in the United States. As powerful entities within the healthcare landscape, they influence each other through a web of financial incentives, lobbying efforts, and strategic negotiations. This connection not only determines the prices consumers pay for medications but also contributes to the rising costs of healthcare as a whole. Patients often find themselves caught in a system where profits take precedence over accessibility, leading to difficult choices and deteriorating health outcomes. Understanding how these two industries interact is essential to uncovering the underlying causes of high drug prices and finding viable paths toward meaningful reform in American healthcare

Impacts on Drug Prices and Overall Healthcare Costs

The relationship between pharmaceutical companies (commonly referred to as Big Pharma) and insurance companies plays a crucial role in determining the cost of medications in the United States. This connection not only influences drug pricing but also has far-reaching implications for the overall cost of healthcare for American consumers. As these two powerful industries interact, their practices contribute to a healthcare system that often prioritizes profit over patient welfare, leading to increased out-of-pocket expenses and barriers to access for essential medications.

The Role of Pharmacy Benefit Managers (PBMs)

Pharmacy Benefit Managers (PBMs) play a pivotal role in the complex relationship between pharmaceutical companies and insurance providers, acting as intermediaries that negotiate drug prices, manage formularies, and establish coverage terms within insurance plans. Positioned as key negotiators, PBMs wield significant influence over the availability and affordability of medications, particularly through their ability to secure rebates from pharmaceutical manufacturers. These rebates are intended to reduce overall drug costs, allowing PBMs to negotiate lower prices on behalf of insurers. However, the reality of these negotiations often diverges from their intended purpose, leading to price distortions that can keep drug costs high for consumers.

One of the main ways PBMs exert influence is by determining which drugs are included in an insurance plan's formulary—the list of medications that are covered, and at what level, by an insurer. To remain on these formularies, pharmaceutical companies frequently agree to substantial rebates, payments made to PBMs in exchange for preferred placement on formulary lists. However, while these rebates lower the initial cost of the drug for PBMs and insurers, they are not consistently passed on to consumers, who may see little or no reduction in the price they pay at the pharmacy counter. Instead, insurers and PBMs often benefit financially from the rebate arrangements, keeping a significant portion of the savings without translating them into lower costs for patients.

The lack of transparency in PBM operations compounds the problem, making it difficult for consumers, healthcare providers, and policymakers to fully understand how drug prices are set and where the rebate dollars ultimately go. In many cases, PBMs do not disclose the details of their rebate negotiations, the size of the discounts obtained, or the extent to which those rebates actually reduce costs for end-users. As a result, consumers and even some healthcare providers are left unaware of how pricing decisions are made, why certain medications are prioritized over others, and whether the cost they're paying reflects the actual market value of the drug (Sullivan et al., 2022).

The opaque nature of PBM practices has attracted increased scrutiny, as critics argue that PBMs prioritize profit over patient affordability, leveraging their market position to maintain high drug prices. Policymakers and advocacy groups have called for greater transparency and regulatory oversight of PBMs to ensure that savings from rebates are shared with consumers. Some proposed solutions include requiring PBMs to disclose rebate amounts and demonstrate how these savings lower out-of-pocket costs for patients. Additionally, legislative efforts have been introduced in Congress to mandate that PBMs pass a larger portion of rebates on to consumers directly, particularly for high-cost medications that place a heavy financial burden on patients.

This section delves into the critical role PBMs play in the pharmaceutical supply chain, examining how their negotiations influence drug pricing and formulary decisions and why their operations have become a focal point in discussions on drug price reform. The influence PBMs hold, coupled with their lack of transparency, underscores the challenges consumers face in accessing affordable medication and highlights the need for reforms that promote clarity and accountability within the healthcare system.

Incentivizing High Drug Prices

The interactions between pharmaceutical companies and insurance providers create incentives that often favor high-cost medications, contributing to the ongoing issue of inflated drug prices. A common mechanism through which these incentives operate is the tiered formulary system that most insurance plans use. In these systems, drugs are categorized into different tiers based on their cost and coverage level, with higher-tier drugs typically incurring higher copayments or coinsurance for patients. While the goal of tiered formularies is to manage costs and encourage the use of more affordable drugs, pharmaceutical companies frequently negotiate to place their products on lower tiers to increase their attractiveness to both patients and healthcare providers. By paying for preferred placement on formularies, high-cost drugs are positioned as more accessible and affordable than they would otherwise be, despite the availability of cheaper alternatives (Kesselheim et al., 2019).

This preferential placement creates an environment where expensive drugs are more likely to be prescribed and used, often without patients being fully informed about lower-cost options that may be just as effective. With high-cost medications more prominently displayed on formularies, patients and providers alike may assume these are the best or only options, leading patients to select these drugs despite their elevated out-of-pocket costs. This can drive up overall healthcare spending as patients are funneled toward higher-priced medications, while insurers benefit from increased premiums and pharmaceutical companies from sustained high prices.

Moreover, this dynamic perpetuates a cycle where high drug prices become normalized, as the prominence of costly drugs on formularies reinforces their place in the market and entrenches pricing practices that maintain high costs. Patients are left bearing the financial burden, with increased copayments and deductibles that contribute to financial strain. Over time, this normalization of high prices discourages the pursuit of more affordable options, as both insurance companies and pharmaceutical manufacturers benefit financially from the status quo.

The entrenchment of high prices in the formulary system also stifles the competition that generics and biosimilars could otherwise provide. Even when more affordable alternatives are available, they are often placed on higher tiers, with insurers and PBMs incentivized to keep high-priced brand-name drugs on the lowest tiers due to the lucrative rebates offered by pharmaceutical companies. This creates a disincentive for healthcare providers to prescribe generics or biosimilars, perpetuating reliance on brand-name medications and delaying the cost-lowering effects of competitive pricing.

This section explores how the interactions between Big Pharma and insurance companies encourage the prioritization of high-cost drugs, examining the effects of tiered formularies, financial incentives, and formulary placement on patient choices and healthcare costs. By highlighting these dynamics, we can better understand the structural factors that drive up drug prices and limit patients' access to affordable treatment options, illustrating the need for greater transparency and reform within the pharmaceutical and insurance industries.

Impact on Overall Healthcare Costs

The connection between Big Pharma and insurance companies extends beyond just drug prices, significantly affecting the overall landscape of healthcare costs in the United States. High drug prices are a key driver behind the escalating premiums and out-of-pocket expenses for consumers, impacting the affordability of healthcare for millions. When insurers absorb the high costs of brand-name and specialty drugs, they often pass these expenses on to consumers in various ways, including higher premiums, increased deductibles, and larger copayments. This trend places a growing financial burden on families and individuals, with many struggling to keep up with the rising costs of their healthcare plans (Fuchs et al., 2022).

The ripple effect of high drug prices is profound, reaching beyond individual expenses to impact health outcomes and the overall effectiveness of the healthcare system. When medications become unaffordable, patients may skip doses, ration their prescriptions, or avoid filling prescriptions entirely, all of which can lead to adverse health outcomes. Chronic conditions that are left untreated or inadequately managed due to cost concerns can worsen over time, leading to more severe health issues that require emergency intervention, hospitalization, or specialized care. These choices—driven by financial necessity rather than medical advice—ultimately place patients at risk and diminish their quality of life.

For healthcare providers, this translates into a heavier burden as they address the complications of untreated or undertreated conditions. Hospitals, clinics, and other facilities frequently absorb the costs associated with providing care for patients who arrive in critical condition due to lack of access to necessary medications. This increased demand for emergency services and intensive care places additional financial strain on healthcare institutions, many of which must divert resources from other essential services to handle the influx of patients with preventable complications. As a result, high drug prices not only affect patients directly but also contribute to higher operating costs for healthcare facilities, creating a feedback loop that drives overall healthcare costs even higher.

The financial implications extend to government programs like Medicare and Medicaid as well. With more beneficiaries requiring advanced treatments due to complications from untreated conditions, these programs experience greater expenditure, putting strain on federal and state budgets. The increased demand on government-funded programs leads to a cycle of rising healthcare costs, which may prompt cuts in other services or increases in taxes to sustain healthcare budgets.

This section examines the cascading effects of high drug prices, exploring how the financial ties between pharmaceutical companies and insurance providers influence the broader healthcare system. By analyzing the interconnectedness of drug prices, insurance premiums, and patient health outcomes, it becomes evident that the high cost of medications affects not just those in need of prescriptions but the sustainability and accessibility of healthcare as a whole in the United States.

The Burden on Taxpayers

The interconnectedness between Big Pharma and insurance companies creates a significant financial burden on taxpayers, particularly as high drug prices limit individuals' access to necessary medications. When patients are unable to afford their prescriptions, they often delay treatment, skip doses, or forego their medications altogether. This lack of access exacerbates health issues, leading many individuals to rely on emergency services and publicly funded healthcare programs like Medicaid and Medicare when their conditions worsen. As a result, taxpayer-funded programs must absorb the rising costs associated with emergency and urgent care visits, creating a substantial drain on government resources.

Medicaid and Medicare, serving as essential safety nets for millions of Americans, are disproportionately impacted by the consequences of unaffordable medications. High drug prices contribute to a cycle in which these programs bear the costs of patients who could have otherwise managed their conditions with affordable prescriptions. This influx of high-cost treatments and emergency interventions strains federal and state budgets, diverting taxpayer dollars that could otherwise be allocated to preventive care, public health initiatives, or infrastructure improvements within the healthcare system.

The economic impact extends further, as the government must continually increase funding for these programs to meet the rising demand for care. Taxpayers, in turn, face indirect costs, as the allocation of government resources increasingly prioritizes short-term solutions—such as covering emergency treatments—over long-term, preventive measures that could reduce overall healthcare spending. High drug prices thus become not only a financial burden on individual patients but also a systemic issue that drains public funds, creating a ripple effect that permeates the broader economy.

Additionally, the strain on publicly funded healthcare programs increases the urgency for systemic reform. The consistent need for taxpayer funding to address high drug costs has led to greater calls for reform, as taxpayers and policymakers alike recognize the unsustainable trajectory of healthcare spending. Advocates argue that reducing drug prices and improving access to affordable medications would alleviate some of the financial pressure on Medicaid and Medicare, enabling these programs to allocate resources more effectively and focus on preventive, patient-centered care rather than reactive, crisis-driven interventions.

This section explores how the interconnectedness of pharmaceutical and insurance companies impacts not only individual patients but the broader economic landscape. By understanding the ways in which high drug prices burden taxpayers and strain public resources, we gain insight into the systemic nature of the issue and the need for healthcare reforms that prioritize affordability, transparency, and sustainability across the healthcare system.

Moving Toward Transparency and Reform

To effectively tackle the challenges posed by the interconnectedness of Big Pharma, insurance companies, and Pharmacy Benefit Managers (PBMs), substantial reforms are necessary to increase transparency, accountability, and consumer protection in the healthcare industry. One of the most pressing needs is to introduce policies that promote clearer pricing structures across the pharmaceutical supply chain. Currently, the lack of transparency around pricing negotiations and rebate agreements obscures the true cost of medications, leaving consumers with little insight into how their out-of-pocket costs are determined. By requiring clearer, standardized pricing disclosures, policymakers can ensure that consumers are better informed about drug costs and are not unduly burdened by hidden fees and markups embedded within insurance and PBM arrangements.

An essential component of reform involves ensuring that the financial benefits of negotiated rebates are passed directly to consumers rather than absorbed by insurers and PBMs. Currently, these entities often retain a significant portion of the rebates offered by pharmaceutical companies to keep specific drugs on formulary lists, resulting in higher drug costs for patients at the pharmacy counter. By mandating that rebates and discounts directly reduce consumer costs, reforms could make prescription medications more affordable, alleviate the financial burden on patients, and increase fairness in the system.

Reducing the outsized influence of pharmaceutical lobbying is also crucial. Big Pharma wields substantial power in shaping healthcare policy through extensive lobbying efforts and campaign contributions. This influence often results in policies that prioritize industry profit over patient welfare, such as laws preventing Medicare from negotiating drug prices or the extension of exclusivity periods for brand-name drugs. By implementing stricter regulations on lobbying practices and campaign finance, policymakers can limit the sway of pharmaceutical interests, ensuring that legislative actions prioritize consumer interests and public health.

Another critical area of reform is fostering competition within the pharmaceutical market. One of the primary ways to achieve this is by expediting the approval processes for generics and biosimilars. Generics and biosimilars introduce competition to the marketplace, often leading to price reductions as more affordable alternatives become available. Streamlining the approval process, reducing exclusivity periods for brand-name drugs, and encouraging the production of biosimilars can help lower prices, increase access, and reduce the dependency on high-cost brand-name medications. This approach would create a more balanced market that promotes affordability and consumer choice.

Addressing the incentives that drive high drug prices and create barriers to access requires a comprehensive approach that considers the systemic issues underpinning the healthcare industry. By reforming the financial incentives that prioritize profit over patient needs, lawmakers can work toward a healthcare system that values equitable access and long-term patient welfare. Such reforms not only have the potential to reduce drug prices but also to make the overall healthcare system more sustainable by easing the financial strain on patients, taxpayers, and government programs like Medicare and Medicaid.

Ultimately, the interconnected relationships among Big Pharma, insurers, and PBMs have created a complex web that significantly influences drug prices and healthcare costs in the United States. By understanding these dynamics, it becomes clear that meaningful reform must address the underlying structures that allow these industries to thrive at the expense of consumers. Only through a commitment to transparency, accountability, and a renewed focus on patient-centered policies can we alleviate the financial burdens associated with high drug prices and build a more equitable healthcare system for all. These reforms are essential steps in creating a system where the primary focus is on promoting public health and ensuring that essential medications are accessible and affordable for every American.

Chapter 14

The Future of Prescription Drug Pricing

The rising cost of prescription drugs in the United States has left patients, policymakers, and healthcare providers grappling with an urgent and complex issue. While recent discussions have brought greater awareness to the issue, meaningful reform remains elusive. As we've explored throughout this book, the U.S. pharmaceutical landscape faces numerous structural, political, and economic challenges that drive high drug prices and hinder access to affordable medications. Drawing lessons from global models and highlighting the collective power of policymakers, healthcare providers, and patients, this conclusion calls for a concerted, multifaceted effort to create a more equitable pharmaceutical system.

Recap of the Main Issues and the Challenges Ahead

The factors driving high drug prices in the U.S. are deeply rooted in the unique structure of its healthcare system. Key issues include the absence of Medicare price negotiations, the prevalence of monopolistic practices such as patent evergreening, and the immense lobbying power of the pharmaceutical industry. Unlike other developed countries, where governments play a central role in price regulation, the U.S. has left pricing largely to market forces, resulting in significant variability and higher costs (Kesselheim et al., 2019). Additionally, the fragmented insurance system and lack of price transparency prevent patients from making informed decisions and place considerable financial burdens on individuals.

The challenges ahead are substantial. Any major reform will require overcoming political opposition, addressing concerns about impacts on innovation, and navigating the powerful lobbying influence of the pharmaceutical industry. Legislative gridlock further complicates the path to reform, as recent policy proposals for Medicare negotiation and price transparency have struggled to gain bipartisan support. The task of lowering drug prices will require sustained effort, creative policy solutions, and a shift in perspective from viewing healthcare as a commodity to recognizing it as a fundamental right. This section summarizes these core issues and highlights the obstacles that remain in creating a sustainable, patient-focused pharmaceutical system.

What America Can Learn from Global Models

The experiences of other countries offer valuable insights into successful strategies for managing drug prices, balancing access, affordability, and innovation through government-led negotiations, price caps, and regulated market entry for generics and biosimilars. Nations like Canada, Australia, and Germany have demonstrated that strategic government intervention can create a pharmaceutical market that serves public health interests without stifling innovation.

Canada's Patented Medicine Prices Review Board (PMPRB), for example, assesses the cost-effectiveness of new drugs and compares them to reference prices from other high-income countries to prevent unjustified price increases. This system ensures that drug prices align with therapeutic value, helping Canadians access essential medications without the excessive costs seen in the U.S. (Morgan et al., 2017). Similarly, the United Kingdom's National Health Service (NHS) negotiates directly with pharmaceutical companies to leverage its centralized purchasing power, securing lower prices that reduce out-of-pocket expenses for patients and keep healthcare expenditures manageable (Kanavos et al., 2011).

The U.S., with its unique blend of public and private insurance, could adapt elements of these international models to create a more affordable drug market. One potential approach is to empower Medicare to negotiate drug prices directly with pharmaceutical companies. By acting as a unified buyer, Medicare could secure substantial cost savings for seniors and taxpayers, mirroring the cost efficiencies achieved by the NHS in the UK. Additionally, implementing price caps for essential drugs—especially those with minimal competition—could provide a safety net against sudden, unregulated price spikes.

The regulated market entry for generics and biosimilars is another strategy that the U.S. could consider. Many countries streamline the approval process for generics and biosimilars to encourage market competition shortly after a drug's patent expires, helping to drive down prices. The U.S. could expedite similar reforms by simplifying regulatory pathways for generics and incentivizing providers to prescribe cost-effective alternatives, making essential treatments more accessible.

Although the U.S. healthcare system is distinct in its structure, the success of these global models underscores the potential impact of government intervention in moderating drug costs. Adapting these approaches could yield significant savings and improve access for American patients without compromising the innovative capacity of the pharmaceutical industry. By examining Canada's pricing evaluations, the UK's centralized negotiation model, and streamlined entry for generics, this section explores how these strategies could shape an affordable, sustainable drug pricing model for the U.S., where patients benefit from essential medications at reasonable costs.

A Call to Action for Policymakers, Healthcare Providers, and Patients

Achieving a sustainable solution to high drug prices in the U.S. requires commitment and action from all stakeholders: policymakers, healthcare providers, and patients themselves. Policymakers must be willing to champion reform efforts that prioritize patient needs over pharmaceutical profits, such as supporting Medicare price negotiations, implementing patent reform, and increasing price transparency (Frank & Ginsburg, 2017). Bipartisan cooperation will be essential to navigate legislative barriers and create policies that balance affordability with innovation.

Healthcare providers also play a critical role in advocating for their patients. By choosing generics when available, participating in patient education on treatment options, and actively supporting policy changes, providers can help mitigate the financial impact of high drug prices on patients. Providers can also partner with organizations like Patients for Affordable Drugs, which advocate for policy changes and support patients in navigating complex pricing and insurance structures (Sachs, 2021).

Patients, too, have a powerful voice. Grassroots movements, public demonstrations, and campaigns can keep the pressure on lawmakers to prioritize reform. Social media, community forums, and advocacy groups offer platforms where patients can share their experiences and demand change. By staying informed, joining advocacy groups, and voting for representatives who prioritize healthcare reform, patients can be pivotal in the push for a more affordable healthcare system. This section underscores the need for collective action, detailing ways in which each stakeholder group can contribute to a more equitable drug pricing landscape.

The future of prescription drug pricing in the United States depends on the collective resolve of policymakers, healthcare providers, and patients to demand and implement transformative change. As explored throughout this book, the high cost of medications in the U.S. is not an isolated issue but one deeply embedded in a complex web of industry practices, regulatory gaps, and financial incentives that prioritize profits over patient access. However, by looking to successful global models, empowering Medicare to negotiate prices, expanding access to generics and biosimilars, and curbing the influence of pharmaceutical lobbying, there is a clear pathway toward a fairer, more affordable system.

While the obstacles are significant, including political gridlock and powerful industry resistance, the urgent need for reform is undeniable. Achieving a sustainable solution will require an unwavering commitment from all stakeholders—policymakers willing to stand against powerful interests, healthcare providers advocating for cost-effective treatment options, and patients uniting to demand transparency and accountability. The journey toward a healthcare system that values patient well-being over profit margins is far from over, but with continued advocacy and informed decision-making, affordable access to essential medications is within reach. The opportunity for lasting change is here; now is the time to act.

Bibliography

Abbott, T., & Vernon, J. A. (2007). The cost of US pharmaceutical price regulation: A financial simulation model of R&D decisions. Journal of Pharmaceutical Finance, Economics & Policy, 16(2), 1-23.

Anderson, G. F., Hussey, P., & Petrosyan, V. (2019). It's still the prices, stupid: Why the US spends so much on health care, and a tribute to Uwe Reinhardt. Health Affairs, 38(1), 87-95. https://doi.org/10.1377/hlthaff.2018.05144

Anderson, G. F., Hussey, P., & Petrosyan, V. (2021). It's still the prices, stupid: Why the U.S. spends so much on health care, and a tribute to Uwe Reinhardt. Health Affairs, 40(4), 567-573.

Biden, J. (2021). Executive Order on Promoting Competition in the American Economy. The White House. Retrieved from https://www.whitehouse.gov.

California Department of Public Health. (2020). CalRx: California's Prescription Drug Initiative. Retrieved from https://www.cdph.ca.gov.

Carpenter, D. (2014). Reputation and power: Organizational image and pharmaceutical regulation at the FDA. Princeton University Press.

Carrier, M. A. (2009). Innovation for the 21st Century: Harnessing the Power of Intellectual Property and Antitrust Law. Oxford University Press.

Carrier, M. A. (2009). Pay for delay: How drug company pay-offs cost consumers billions. Health Affairs, 28(1), w109-w118. https://doi.org/10.1377/hlthaff.28.1.w109

Centers for Medicare & Medicaid Services. (2022). National health expenditure data. Retrieved from https://www.cms.gov

Chaudhuri, S., Goldberg, P. K., & Jia, P. (2006). Estimating the effects of global patent protection in pharmaceuticals: A case study of quinolones in India. The American Economic Review, 96(5), 1477-1514.

Cohen, J. C., Mrazek, M., & Hawkins, L. (2010). "Corruption and pharmaceuticals: Strengthening good governance to improve access." In Global Corruption Report: Corruption and Health, ed. Transparency International. Routledge.

Collins, S. R., Gunja, M. Z., Doty, M. M., & Beutel, S. (2018). How well does insurance coverage protect consumers from health care costs?. The Commonwealth Fund.

Cubanski, J., & Damico, A. (2019). Closing the Medicare Part D coverage gap: Trends, recent changes, and what's ahead. Kaiser Family Foundation.

Dieguez, G., Alston, M., Chu, B., & Nelson, L. (2020). Prescription Drug Spending: Growth and Contributing Factors. Milliman Research Report.

DiMasi, J. A., Grabowski, H. G., & Hansen, R. W. (2016). Innovation in the pharmaceutical industry: New estimates of R&D costs. Journal of Health Economics, 47, 20-33. https://doi.org/10.1016/j.jhealeco.2016.01.012

Donohue, J. M., Cevasco, M., & Rosenthal, M. B. (2007). A decade of direct-to-consumer advertising of prescription drugs. The New England Journal of Medicine, 357(7), 673-681. https://doi.org/10.1056/NEJMsa070502

Duckett, S., & Willcox, S. (2015). The Australian Healthcare System. Oxford University Press.

Dylst, P., Vulto, A., & Simoens, S. (2013). Demand-side policies to encourage the use of generic medicines: An overview. Expert

Review of Pharmacoeconomics & Outcomes Research, 13(1), 59-72.

European Commission. (2022). Pharmaceutical Strategy for Europe. Retrieved from https://ec.europa.eu

FDA. (2022). Milestones in U.S. food and drug law history. Retrieved from https://www.fda.gov

Feldman, R. (2018). May your drug price be evergreen. Journal of Law and the Biosciences, 5(3), 590-647.

Frank, R. G., & Ginsburg, P. B. (2017). Pharmaceuticals and public health: Prospects for a new policy. Health Affairs, 36(1), 159-166.

Frosch, D. L., Krueger, P. M., Hornik, R. C., Cronholm, P. F., & Barg, F. K. (2007). Creating demand for prescription drugs: A content analysis of television direct-to-consumer advertising. Annals of Family Medicine, 5(1), 6-13.

Fuchs, V. R., Garber, A. M., & Hsu, J. (2022). High and Rising Drug Prices: Causes and Consequences. *Health Affairs*, 41(3), 345-354. https://doi.org/10.1377/hlthaff.2021.01512

Gleeson, D., Lopert, R., & Reid, P. (2019). The high price of "free" trade: U.S. trade agreements and access to medicines. Journal of Law, Medicine & Ethics, 47(1), 99-115.

Geyman, J. P. (2015). How Obamacare Is Unsustainable: Why We Need a Single-Payer Solution for All Americans. Copernicus Healthcare.

Grabowski, H. G., Long, G., & Mortimer, R. (2016). Recent trends in brand-name and generic drug competition. Health Affairs, 35(5), 924-931.

Greene, J. A., & Riggs, K. R. (2019). Why is there no generic insulin? Historical origins of a modern problem. New England Journal of Medicine, 372(12), 1171-1175.

Hemminki, E. (2010). The regulation of pharmaceutical advertising in the European Union. Health Policy, 57(4), 305-314.

Hemphill, C. S., & Sampat, B. N. (2012). Evergreening, patent challenges, and effective market life in pharmaceuticals. Journal of Health Economics, 31(2), 327-339. https://doi.org/10.1016/j.jhealeco.2012.01.004

Hirsch, D. (2021). The origins of pharmaceutical giants: A brief history of American drug companies. Journal of Health and Bioethics, 22(1), 44-59.

Holman, L. (2022). The FDA and Moderna's cosy relationship: how lax rules enable a revolving door. *The BMJ*, 383, p2486.

Huang, J., & Catlin, M. (2021). The impact of Medicare Part D on prescription drug prices and insurance coverage. Journal of Health Economics, 74, 102377.

Hutt, P. B., & Merrill, R. A. (2020). Food and drug law: Cases and materials. Foundation Press.

Ikegami, N., & Anderson, G. F. (2012). In Japan, all-payer rate setting under tight government control has proved to be an effective approach to containing costs. Health Affairs, 31(5), 1049-1056.

IQVIA. (2023). 2022 U.S. Pharmaceutical Market Performance. IQVIA Institute for Human Data Science.

Kaiser Family Foundation (KFF). (2019). Prescription drugs. Retrieved from https://www.kff.org

Kanavos, P., Ferrario, A., Vandoros, S., & Anderson, G. F. (2011). Higher US Branded Drug Prices and Spending Compared to Other Countries May Stem Partly from Quick Uptake of New Drugs. Health Affairs, 32(4), 753-761.

Kesselheim, A. S., Avorn, J., & Sarpatwari, A. (2011). The High Cost of Prescription Drugs in the United States: Origins and Prospects for Reform. JAMA, 316(8), 858-871.

Kesselheim, A. S., Avorn, J., & Sarpatwari, A. (2018). The high cost of prescription drugs in the United States: Origins and prospects for reform. JAMA, 316(8), 858-871. https://doi.org/10.1001/jama.2018.5601

Kesselheim, A. S., Avorn, J., & Sarpatwari, A. (2019). The high cost of prescription drugs in the United States: Origins and prospects for reform. Journal of the American Medical Association, 316(8), 858-871.

Kesselheim, A. S., & Avorn, J. (2021). The high cost of prescription drugs in the United States: Origins and prospects for reform. JAMA, 316(8), 858-871.

Lexchin, J., & Mintzes, B. (2002). Direct-to-consumer advertising of prescription drugs: The evidence says no. Journal of Public Policy & Marketing, 21(2), 194-201.

Mazzucato, M. (2018). The Value of Everything: Making and Taking in the Global Economy. PublicAffairs.

Mintzes, B. (2012). Disease mongering in drug promotion: do governments have a regulatory role? PLoS Medicine, 9(5), e1001211.

Mintzes, B., Mangin, D., Hayes, L., Coughlan, E., & Rachlis, B. (2019). Drug promotion and prescribing in Australia, the United States, and Canada: A qualitative study of the experiences and views of pharmacists, physicians, and consumers. Journal of Public Health Policy, 40(1), 106-124. https://doi.org/10.1057/s41271-018-015

Morgan, S. G., Bathula, H. S., & Moon, S. (2017). Pricing of pharmaceuticals is becoming a major challenge for health systems. BMJ, 358, j3500. https://doi.org/10.1136/bmj.j3500

Moynihan, R., Heath, I., & Henry, D. (2002). Selling sickness: The pharmaceutical industry and disease mongering. British Medical Journal, 324(7342), 886-891.

Oberlander, J. (2010). The Political History of Medicare. The Journal of Law, Medicine & Ethics, 38(4), 795-798.

OECD. (2022). Health at a glance 2022: OECD indicators. OECD Publishing. http Staton, T. (2021). AbbVie's Humira patent thicket faces new scrutiny as biosimilars loom. *Fierce Pharma*.s://doi.org/10.1787/health_glance-2022-en

OpenSecrets. (2022). Pharmaceuticals/Health Products: Money to Congress. Retrieved from https://www.opensecrets.org.

Ornstein, C., & Weber, T. (2018). Big Pharma's Revolving Door: The Back-and-Forth Flow of Officials Between Drug Firms and Federal Agencies. ProPublica. Retrieved from https://www.propublica.org.

Outterson, K. (2005). Pharmaceutical arbitrage: balancing access and innovation in international prescription drug markets. Yale Journal of Health Policy, Law, and Ethics, 5(1), 193-290.

Proctor, C. (2021). Big Pharma Lobbying Dollars Target Medicare Pricing Reform. Forbes. Retrieved from https://www.forbes.com.

Rosenthal, M. B., Berndt, E. R., Donohue, J. M., Epstein, A. M., & Frank, R. G. (2016). Demand effects of recent changes in prescription drug promotion. Frontiers in Health Policy Research, 6, 1-26.

Sachs, R. (2021). Prescription Drug Pricing: The Role of Federal Policy and Industry Innovation. National Academies Press.

Sarnak, D. O., Squires, D., Bishop, S., & Anderson, C. (2017). Paying for prescription drugs around the world: Why is the US an outlier?

The Commonwealth Fund. Retrieved from https://www.commonwealthfund.org

Schwartz, L. M., & Woloshin, S. (2019). Medical marketing in the United States, 1997-2016. Journal of the American Medical Association, 321(1), 80-96.

Sullivan, M., Nuss, D., & Oscherwitz, T. (2022). Understanding the Role of Pharmacy Benefit Managers in Drug Pricing. *American Journal of Managed Care*, 28(2), 68-73. https://doi.org/10.37765/ajmc.2022.10409

Sweeny, K. (2014). The impact of public and private sector partnerships on Australia's Pharmaceutical Benefits Scheme. Australian Health Review, 38(4), 397-403.

Tabernero, J., Vyas, M., Giuliani, R., Arnold, D., & Cardoso, F. (2017). Biosimilars: A position paper of the European Society for Medical Oncology, with particular reference to oncology prescribers. ESMO Open, 1(6), e000142.

Taylor, D., & Gomez, H. (2019). The Role of the Pharmaceutical Industry in U.S. Health Care Reform. American Journal of Public Health, 109(8), 1097-1103.

Taylor, C., Steagall, A., & Driessen, E. (2019). The influence of pharmaceutical industry spending on drug pricing reform in the United States. Journal of Health Politics, Policy and Law, 44(6), 907-932. https://doi.org/10.1215/03616878-7806633

Toop, L., Richards, D., Dowell, A., Tilyard, M., Fraser, T., Arroll, B., & Jackson, R. (2003). Direct-to-consumer advertising of prescription drugs in New Zealand: For health or for profit? Journal of the New Zealand Medical Association, 116(1180).

Vogler, S., Paris, V., & Ferrario, A. (2017). How can pricing and reimbursement policies improve affordable access to medicines?

Lessons from European countries. Bulletin of the World Health Organization, 95(11), 720-727.

Wouters, O. J., Kanavos, P. G., & McKee, M. (2020). Comparing generic drug markets in Europe and the United States: Prices, volumes, and spending. The Milbank Quarterly, 98(1), 38-65. https://doi.org/10.1111/1468-0009.12430

Zuckerman, D. M., & Browne, T. (2017). "21st Century Cures Act: The Good, the Bad, and the Ugly." The BMJ, 358, j4057.

About the Author

Dr. Douglas B. Sims is a distinguished environmental soil scientist with more than 30 years of experience in the environmental consulting industry. He holds a bachelor's and master's degree from the University of Nevada, Las Vegas, and earned his PhD from Kingston University London, specializing in environmental science and sustainable land management. In 2011, Dr. Sims shifted from the private sector to academia, joining the College of Southern Nevada (CSN) as an environmental science educator. His expertise and vision led to his appointment as Dean of the School of Science, Engineering, and Mathematics at CSN, where he has been pivotal in aligning academic programs with industry standards, equipping students for careers in science and engineering.

Dr. Sims has also been an active researcher throughout his career, publishing extensively in peer-reviewed journals on soil remediation and environmental contamination. His contributions have significantly influenced both academic discourse and practical applications in environmental science. Known for his commitment to education, Dr. Sims has played a key role in shaping the future of environmental science by fostering student success and developing impactful programs.

Beyond his professional accomplishments, Dr. Sims is a keen observer of the complexities in American politics and social dynamics. He holds a particular interest in the high cost of pharmaceuticals in the U.S. and the political paradoxes within the Republican and Democratic parties. His ability to connect scientific inquiry with broader societal and political challenges lends a unique perspective on these pressing issues. Married to his college sweetheart since the mid-1990s, Dr. Sims and his wife have raised two children, fostering a family grounded in curiosity, education, and shared values.

Glossary of Key Terms

Biologics: Complex drugs derived from living organisms, often used to treat conditions like cancer and autoimmune diseases. Biologics require unique manufacturing processes and are generally more expensive than traditional drugs.

Biosimilars: Highly similar versions of biologic drugs, intended to provide comparable therapeutic effects at a lower cost. Biosimilars are common in countries with regulated drug pricing systems.

Direct-to-Consumer (DTC) Advertising: Marketing aimed directly at consumers, which is legal only in the U.S. and New Zealand, allowing pharmaceutical companies to promote prescription drugs to the public.

Evergreening: A strategy where pharmaceutical companies make minor modifications to a drug to extend its patent life, delaying the entry of generic or biosimilar competitors.

Generic Drugs: Chemically identical versions of brand-name drugs that become available once patents expire, typically offered at lower prices.

Medicare Part D: A federal program that provides prescription drug coverage to Medicare beneficiaries, but currently does not allow Medicare to negotiate drug prices directly.

Patent Cliff: The expiration of a drug patent, which allows generic versions to enter the market and often results in a significant drop in the drug's price.

Pharmaceutical Benefits Scheme (PBS): Australia's government-funded program that negotiates drug prices, making medications affordable for Australian citizens.

Price Negotiation: A process in which a government or large buyer bargains with pharmaceutical companies to set drug prices, used in many countries to control costs.

Reference Pricing: A pricing system where a country uses the cost of a drug in other countries as a benchmark to set domestic prices.

Legislative Timeline

Key laws impacting drug prices in the U.S. and EU

United States

- **1984**: *Hatch-Waxman Act* – Facilitated the approval of generic drugs, creating a faster pathway for generics to enter the market while preserving some exclusivity for brand-name drugs (U.S. FDA, 2018).
- **2003**: *Medicare Prescription Drug, Improvement, and Modernization Act* – Established Medicare Part D, providing drug coverage for seniors but prohibiting Medicare from negotiating prices.
- **2010**: *Affordable Care Act (ACA)* – Introduced provisions aimed at closing the Medicare Part D coverage gap and promoting competition in the pharmaceutical market.
- **2019**: *CREATES Act* – Designed to prevent anti-competitive practices that delay generic drug entry, enabling faster access to affordable alternatives.
- **2021**: *Executive Order on Promoting Competition in the American Economy* – Proposed Medicare negotiations on certain high-cost drugs, marking an attempt at federal-level price control (Biden, 2021).

European Union

- **1992**: *Transparency Directive* – Mandated transparency in drug pricing across EU countries, establishing criteria for fair price setting and enabling price comparisons across member states (European Commission, 2019).
- **2004**: *EU Clinical Trials Directive* – Standardized the drug approval process across member states, balancing access to innovative drugs with patient safety.

- **2009**: *Biologics Price Competition and Innovation Act* – Aimed to increase access to affordable biologics, allowing the EU to approve biosimilars at a faster rate than in the U.S.
- **2017**: *HTA Regulation Proposal* – Called for more collaboration among EU countries on health technology assessments, supporting fairer pricing and accessibility for innovative treatments (European Medicines Agency, 2020).

www.ingramcontent.com/pod-product-compliance
Lightning Source LLC
Chambersburg PA
CBHW070637030426
42337CB00020B/4059